UNDERSTANDING DEVELOPMENT AND DISORDER IN CANTONESE USING LANGUAGE SAMPLE ANALYSIS

Understanding Development and Disorder in Cantonese Using Language Sample Analysis brings together 20 years of research on typical development and development language disorder (DLD) in Cantonese.

This book begins with a succinct overview of Cantonese, which is a popular variety of Chinese, a Sino-Tibetan language. The second chapter describes a new framework of the *Grammatical Analysis of Cantonese Samples* (GACS), which was developed on the basis of functionalist and usage-based theories of language and language development. The third chapter reports on a quantitative analysis, as well as a qualitative description of the development of Cantonese in preschool children using the GACS framework. The book ends with a chapter that presents the linguistic profile of a Cantonese-speaking child with DLD. It also illustrates how to make decisions on intervention targets on the basis of the grammatical and error analysis. The book provides a timely and important addition to the typological diversity of studies in both child language development and disorder.

This book is informative for students and practitioners of speech and language therapy, students in early childhood education and Chinese linguistics and researchers in child language development and disorders.

Anita Mei-Yin Wong is an associate professor in the discipline of speech pathology, Faculty of Medicine and Health, University of Sydney, Australia.

UNDERSTANDING DEVELOPMENT AND DISORDER IN CANTONESE USING LANGUAGE SAMPLE ANALYSIS

Anita Mei-Yin Wong

Routledge
Taylor & Francis Group
LONDON AND NEW YORK

Designed cover image: Anita Mei-Yin Wong

First published 2023
by Routledge
4 Park Square, Milton Park, Abingdon, Oxon OX14 4RN

and by Routledge
605 Third Avenue, New York, NY 10158

Routledge is an imprint of the Taylor & Francis Group, an informa business

British Library Cataloguing-in-Publication Data
A catalogue record for this book is available from the British Library

Library of Congress Cataloging-in-Publication Data
Names: Wong, Anita M-Y., author.
Title: Understanding development and disorder in Cantonese using language sample analysis / Anita Mei-Yin Wong.
Description: New York : Routledge, 2023. | Includes bibliographical references.
Identifiers: LCCN 2022025291 (print) | LCCN 2022025292 (ebook) | ISBN 9780367424183 (hardback) | ISBN 9780367424190 (paperback) | ISBN 9780367824013 (ebook)
Subjects: LCSH: Language disorders in children—China. | Chinese language—Grammar. | Chinese language—Acquisition.
Classification: LCC RJ496.L35 W65 2023 (print) | LCC RJ496.L35 (ebook) | DDC 618.92/85500951—dc23/eng/20220629
LC record available at https://lccn.loc.gov/2022025291
LC ebook record available at https://lccn.loc.gov/2022025292

ISBN: 978-0-367-42418-3 (hbk)
ISBN: 978-0-367-42419-0 (pbk)
ISBN: 978-0-367-82401-3 (ebk)

DOI: 10.4324/9780367824013

Typeset in Bembo
by Apex CoVantage, LLC

I dedicate this book to our parents, Mr. Shing-Fat Wong (1921–1994) and Mrs. Ping Mak-Wong (1931–2006), who gave me a happy start on this life journey, and to my sisters and brother, Ms. Millie Mi-Lee Wong, Ms. Winnie May-Ching Wong, Ms. Brenda Mee-Yung Wong and Mr. Gal Shu-Kei Wong, for their loving company from day one! I thank God for them all!

CONTENTS

PREFACE

I grew up learning Cantonese as my home language. I did not have a choice, but I do wonder once in a while, "What if I did?" Most children did not have a choice on their first language(s) either. We all learn whatever language(s) are in our environment. What intrigues me is that we are all successful in learning at least one home language, although some are better at it than others.

There are about 7,100 different languages in the world (Simons, 2022). In a recent comprehensive survey on the number of languages reported in the four main journals of child language acquisition, Kidd and Garcia (2022) reported that there is a strong Indo-European bias in the published articles from 1974 to 2020. Of the 2,827 articles included in the survey, 54% were on English, and 30% were on the other 38 languages in the Indo-European family. Only the remaining 16% were on languages from other language families. In the field of child language disorders, my educated guess is that there is a similar lack of typological diversity in published journal articles. Datasets that are skewed can have a negative impact on theory building in both fields.

Mandarin and Cantonese are two varieties of Chinese that belong to the Sino-Tibetan family of languages. Among all the non-Indo-European languages, Mandarin follows Hebrew as the second most studied language in the field of child language acquisition, with 83 published articles. Cantonese, with 28 published articles, comes sixth on the list, after Japanese, Finnish and Korean (Kidd & Garcia, 2022). The Yue dialect, of which Cantonese is a member, is ranked nineteenth on the list of the world's most spoken languages (Ethnologue, 2022).

This book is written for speech-language therapists, or speech-language pathologists in some professional contexts; child language researchers; and early childhood educators who have a clinical and/or research interest in learning more about language development and developmental language disorder in young Cantonese-speaking children. The aims of this book are

1. to provide an overview of Cantonese grammar, which is the end state of a child's language development,
2. to describe a new framework for the grammatical analysis of Cantonese conversational samples,
3. to validate MLU100 and a summative score obtained from the grammatical analysis of a language sample as measures of grammatical development in Cantonese,
4. to provide a qualitative overview of grammatical development by age group and on individual children,
5. to give an overview of the linguistic characteristics of developmental language disorder (DLD) in Cantonese,
6. to discuss in detail the linguistic profile of a Cantonese-speaking child with DLD, and last but not least,
7. to illustrate how to make decisions on intervention goals on the basis of a language sample analysis.

It is my hope that this book will be an impetus for more theoretical and clinical research on developmental language disorder in Cantonese and in Chinese in general.

This book is a celebration of my 20-some years of classroom teaching, clinical education, research, and engagement in professional and public education at the BSc speech and hearing sciences program at the University of Hong Kong. There I learned from my mentors and colleagues and many of our visiting scholars. I also learned with my postgraduate students, my undergraduate honors thesis and final-year project students, and my research associates. Among them, my colleague and EdD student Dr. Cecilia Wing-Sze Au deserves special mention. These were 20-some good years because of you all.

This book is a belated gift to my friend Professor Stephanie Stokes from an intellectual journey that began in 1994 when she bought me the first edition of the book *Cantonese: A Comprehensive Grammar* by Professor Stephen Matthews and Professor Virginia Yip for Christmas. Stephanie's curiosity about language development and language disorders in Cantonese has inspired my work and that of many of our students. Professor Matthews and Professor Yip's comprehensive book, currently in its second edition, is seminal for anyone interested in learning about Cantonese. I am grateful to Steve for his advice on the early versions of the grammatical analysis framework.

I would not have come this far without the supervisors of my postdoc years, Professor Paul Fletcher, Professor Stephanie Stokes and Professor Laurence Leonard. I had the greatest opportunity any fresh PhD could ask for: working on a NIH-funded project on morphosyntactic deficits in Cantonese-speaking children with specific language impairment, the more common term for DLD at the time. Paul, Stephanie and Larry showed me how to study DLD in Cantonese from a cross-linguistic perspective.

This book began with the development of a framework of grammatical analysis. The framework went through several versions, and each version was validated thorough an analysis of language samples. The first version was developed in 2011 by my BSc honors student Ms. Emily Ka-Hei Wan. At the time, it was called *An Index of Syntax Development* (ISD). With the support of the undergraduate research fellowship scheme, Ms. Jessica Man-Wai Lo came up with a revised version in 2015. In 2019, we invited Dr. Candice Chi-Hang Cheung, a Chinese syntactician, to review and further develop the framework with us. The framework was subsequently renamed *The Grammatical Analysis of Cantonese Samples* (GACS). I thank Candice, Jessica and Emily for joining me as co-authors of Chapter 2 of this book. They were all amazing to work with. I thank the Faculty Research Fund for providing funding support for Jessica and Emily to reanalyze the language samples using the GACS framework. I thank my students Ms. Kinny Kin-Ling Yeung and Mr. Darryl Lok-Hin Chan, who helped identify the age of emergence and the age of productive use for the GACS items from the analyzed data. I also thank Professor Tom Klee, whose work on language sample analysis provided useful signposts throughout my book journey.

I would like to thank Paul, Larry and Steve for their review of selected chapters of this book; Mr. Stephen Parsons for his editorial review; and my student Mr. Chris Pak-Lam Lee for formatting all the Cantonese examples provided in Jyutping. All errors that remain are mine. I thank Ms. Iola Ashby and Ms. Andrea Hartill at the Routledge editorial office for seeing the book to its completion. Last but not least, I thank Mr. E-den Mok for teaching me Chinese water ink painting in the past three and a half years. It has been a journey into beauty of the eyes and the mind. The cover of this book was a milestone of that journey.

I will close this preface with the title of the first Elizabeth Bates Lecture given by my MSc academic advisor at Indiana University and my PhD supervisor at the University of British Columbia, Professor Judith Johnston, at the 25th Symposium on Research in Child Language Disorders in 2005. The title is "Fearless and Bold in Following Ideas Wherever They Lead." My ideas are now taking me to the University of Sydney, where I will learn about language development and disorders in Cantonese-speaking children in a different cultural and linguistic milieu. I look forward to seeing what is around the corner.

Anita Mei-Yin Wong
March 2022

1

A GRAMMATICAL OVERVIEW OF CANTONESE

1.1 Introduction

The Chinese language has seven major dialect groups, which are spoken in different geographical areas of China. As a member of the Yue dialect group, Cantonese is spoken in the southern provinces of Guangdong and Guangxi. With over 75 million native speakers (Encyclopedia Britannica, n.d.) in China and in many Chinese communities overseas, including Singapore, Malaysia, Vietnam, Australia and Canada, Cantonese is the most prestigious spoken form of Chinese after Mandarin (Li, 2006; Matthews & Yip, 2011). The Yue dialect is ranked 19th on the list of the world's most spoken languages (Ethnologue, 2022). Mandarin, however, is the largest dialect group in the Chinese language and the most spoken language in the world (Ethnologue, 2022). Mandarin is the basis on which Putonghua, the standard official language of Chinese, was developed. Cantonese and Mandarin are not mutually intelligible, and they also differ in vocabulary and some aspects of grammar. Despite these differences, speakers of Cantonese and Mandarin share and use the same written form of Chinese.

In this chapter, we will present a brief overview of Cantonese, with a focus on morphology and syntax. The goal is to provide a foundation for understanding the framework for analyzing children's conversational samples, which will be presented in Chapter 2. The structure of the overview follows that of Shi and Huang's (2016) chapter on Chinese syntax and Zhan and Bai's (2016) chapter on sentence types. The content of the overview is heavily drawn from Matthews and Yip (2011). Readers may also refer to Cheung (2007) and Tang (2015) for further descriptive details about Cantonese. In situations in which the description is broadly applicable to Chinese, we refer to it as such but give examples in Cantonese. While we will not compare Cantonese with English, we assume that our readers have some basic knowledge of the linguistic description of English.

DOI: 10.4324/9780367824013-1

In this book, we use the Jyutping Romanization System published by the Linguistic Society of Hong Kong (1997) to represent Cantonese syllables. Cantonese examples are presented in the format shown in the example. Note that the first letter of words or phrases on the gloss line is not capitalized. Abbreviations used on the gloss line for function words are listed on page 128. On the translation line, optional nominal elements in Cantonese that can be omitted in context are in parentheses. Complete sentences end with a punctuation mark.

Example

Characters:	*我學咗水墨畫三年有多喇。*
Romanization:	*ngo5 hok6 zo2 seoi2 mak6 waa2 saam1 nin4 jau5do1 laa3*
Gloss:	I learn ASP water ink picture three year excess SFP
Translation:	(I have been learning water-ink painting for more than three years.)

1.2 Lexical tones, morphemes and words

Most Cantonese morphemes are monosyllabic, such as *食 sik6* [eat]. Similar to other varieties of Chinese, Cantonese is a tonal language, meaning that each syllable carries a pitch pattern (level, rising or falling). A change in the pitch pattern of the syllable alters the meaning of the morpheme. For example, the syllables *食 sik6* [eat] and *色 sik1* [color], with one carrying the low level tone 6 and one carrying the high level tone 1, are two different morphemes. There are six lexical tones in Cantonese, and in the Jyutping Romanization System, the tone is represented by a numeral at the end of each syllable.

Many Cantonese words, however, are disyllabic and bimorphemic. These disyllabic words are formed by affixation (e.g., *男仔 naam4zai2* 'boy-little' [little boy]), reduplication (e.g., *波波 bo1bo1* 'ball-ball' [ball]) or compounding (e.g., *傷心 soeng1sam1* 'hurt-heart' [sad]). Compounding is the most productive word-forming process of the three strategies (Packard, 2000). The two morphemes of a word compound may reflect syntactic or semantic relations like subject-predicate (e.g., *頭痛 tau4tung3* 'head-ache' [headache]). The relation of the two morphemes in compounds cannot always be determined, especially in compounds that are highly lexicalized. One example is *孤寒 gu1hon4* 'alone-cool' [stingy]. Some disyllabic words (e.g., *的士 dik1si2* [taxi]) and most polysyllabic words (e.g., *士多啤梨 si6do1be1lei2* [strawberry]) are loan words, in which there are no syntactic or semantic relations between the morphemes. For more details on the structure of words in Cantonese, refer to Tang (2015).

1.3 Word classes

Word classes, also known as parts of speech or syntactic categories, are not overtly marked in Chinese. For example, the word *幫手 bong1sau2* 'help-hand' is a noun in the first sentence [1], but a verb in the second sentence [2]. Although they are not straightforward, Chinese word classes can be determined on the basis of distributional information (Fung, 2009). For example, 幫手 *bong1sau2* in [1] is a noun because it is modified by a classifier, and it is a verb in [2] because it is modified by an adverb.

[1] 我個幫手未嚟呀。
ngo5 go3 bong1sau2 mei6 lei4 aa3
I CL help-hand not-yet come SFP
(My helper has not come yet.)

[2] 你可唔可以即刻幫手整個蛋糕呀？
nei5 ho2-m4-ho2ji5 zik1hak1 bong1sau2 zing2 go3 daan6gou1 aa3
you can-not-can immediately help-hand make CL cake SFP
(Can you help make a cake right away?)

Another example of polysemous forms is the word 俾 *bei2* (Wong, 2004). It can be a verb meaning "to give" or "to allow." It can also be used as a preposition to indicate "to" or "for." Cues that are used to identify the part of speech of polysemous forms can sometimes be implicit.

Chinese includes these word classes: numerals, classifiers, nouns, pronouns, adjectives, verbs, aspect markers, verbal particles, adverbs, prepositions, postpositions or localizers, conjunctions, sentence-final particles, interjections and onomatopoeia. In this section, we highlight the meaning and syntactic properties of the Cantonese word classes as described in Matthews and Yip (2011), focusing on features that are of special interest to English readers who are not too familiar with Chinese.

Numerals and classifiers

The numeral precedes countable nouns, and a classifier appears between the numeral and the noun. The choice of classifiers for countable nouns is often determined by the properties of the nouns. For example, the classifier 隻 *zek3* is used with nouns referring to animals (e.g., dog in [3]), and the classifier 枝 *zi1* refers to long and relatively hard objects (e.g., tree branch). In addition to referring to countable nouns, Cantonese classifiers (e.g., 斤 *gan1* [catty]) also indicate quantities of mass nouns as in [4]. Classifiers are grammatically obligatory when a demonstrative (e.g., 呢 *nei1* [this], 嗰 *go2* [that]) or a numeral is used. The demonstrative, the numeral and the classifier appear before the head noun in the order mentioned as illustrated in [5]. Classifiers also function as markers in possessive constructions as in [6] and relative clauses as in [7]. Note that in Chinese, the relative clause, like other modifying phrases, comes before the head noun.

[3] 三隻狗
saam1 zek3 gau2
three CL dog
(three dogs)

[4] *一斤糖*
jat1 gan1 tong4
one CL sugar
(one catty of sugar)

[5] *嗰三隻狗*
go2 saam1 zek3 gau2
that three CL dog
(those three dogs)

[6] *爸爸對鞋*
baa4baa1 deoi3 haai4
daddy CL shoe
(Daddy's pair of shoes)

[7] *戴耳環個女人*
daai3 ji5waan2 go3 neoi5jan2
wear earring CL woman
(the woman who wears earrings)

Nouns and pronouns

Nouns in Chinese are not marked for number or gender. Definiteness is not indicated by articles equivalent to *a* or *the*, but by the position of the [classifier + noun] phrase relative to the verb. In [8], the [classifier + noun] phrase appearing before the predicate refers to a definite car, whereas the post-verbal phrase in [9] encodes either a definite or an indefinite referent. Unlike nouns, personal pronouns have distinct plural forms, marked by the suffix *哋 dei6* (*我 ngo5* [I], *我哋 ngo5dei6* [we], *你 nei5* [you], *你哋 nei5dei6* [you (plural)], *佢 keoi5* [s/he] or [it], *佢哋 keoi5dei6* [they]). Note that the same pronoun, *佢 keoi5*, is used for the different genders.

[8] *架車好靚。*
gaa3 ce1 hou2 leng3
CL car very pretty
(The car looks very nice.)

[9] *我聽日去買架車。*
ngo5 ting1jat6 heoi3 maai5 gaa3 ce1
I tomorrow go buy CL car
(I will go buy a/the car tomorrow.)

Adjectives and verbs

Adjectives and verbs in Chinese share quite a few syntactic properties, thus making it difficult to draw a distinction between the two in some contexts. For examples, both verbs and adjectives can take aspect markers (e.g., *食咗 sik6 zo2* [have eaten], *靚咗 leng3 zo2* [have become prettier]) and verbal particles (e.g., *飲晒 jam2 saai3* [drink up], *乾晒 gon1 saai3* [all dry]). Some grammarians will argue that Chinese verbs and adjectives form one single category of predicates.

Aspect markers and verbal particles

Cantonese words do not change in form, given the absence of inflectional morphemes for marking person, gender, case, number (except for pronouns), tense or mood. There are, however, bound morphemes (e.g., the perfective aspect marker *咗 zo2*, the progressive aspect marker *緊 gan2*) that appear after the predicate to indicate time relations. See [10] for an illustration. These aspect markers are basically grammatically optional. In other words, a sentence with a verb that is not followed by an aspect marker is not considered a violation of Cantonese grammar. An aspect marker, however, expresses the speaker's viewpoint on a situation. If a speaker chooses not to put in an aspect marker after the predicate, s/he has taken on a neutral viewpoint, as in [11], which can make the sentence sound incomplete.

[10] *佢彈緊琴。*
keoi5 taan4 gan2 kam4
s/he play ASP piano
(S/he is playing the piano.)

[11] *佢彈琴。*
keoi5 taan4 kam4
s/he play piano
(S/he plays the piano.)

In addition to the eight aspect markers, Cantonese has a rich set of verbal particles for indicating result, directions, quantifying and adversative functions. In [12], the resultative particle *好 hou2* [finish] follows the verb *煮 zyu2* [cook] to denote completion. Some of the verbal particles (e.g., *爛 laan6* [broken] in [13]) can appear independently in other contexts as verbs or adjectives (e.g., [14])

[12] *姐姐煮好啲布甸喇。*
ze4ze1 zyu2 hou2 di1 bou3din1 laa3
older-sister cook PRT CL pudding SFP
(The older sister finished cooking the pudding.)

[13] *唔好整爛個杯呀！*
m4hou2 zing2 laan6 go3 bui1 aa3
do-not make PRT CL cup SFP
(Don't break the cup!)

[14] *個杯爛咗。*
go3 bui1 laan6 zo2
CL cup broken ASP
(The cup is broken.)

Sometimes it is hard to make a distinction between some aspect markers and verbal particles because they have very subtle differences in meaning. In [15] the perfective aspect marker *咗 zo2* emphasizes that the result of the event holds at the time of speaking. On the other hand, the resultative particle *到 dou2* [indicating ability] in [16] focuses on the successful completion of the event.

[15] *爸爸開咗道門喇。*
baa4baa1 hoi1 zo2 dou6 mun4 laa3
daddy open ASP CL door SFP
(Daddy has opened the door.)

[16] *爸爸開到道門喇。*
baa4baa1 hoi1 dou2 dou6 mun4 laa3
daddy open PRT CL door SFP
(Daddy successfully opened the door.)

Having said this, aspect markers and verbal particles do differ in syntactic properties. The potential particle *得 dak1* [can] and the negative *唔m4* [not] can go between the verb and the verbal particle as in [17], but not between the verb and the aspect marker.

[17] *佢食得晒啲餅。*
keoi5 sik6 dak1 saai3 di1 beng2 gaa3
s/he eat PRT PRT CL biscuit SFP
(S/he can eat all the biscuits.)

In fact, verbal particles can be combined with aspect markers as in [18], and several verbal particles can also appear together to modify the verb as in [19]. These sentences illustrate how productive verbal particles can be in the modification of the verb phrase.

[18] *啲餅整好咗喇。*
di1 beng2 zing2 hou2 zo2 laa3
CL biscuit make PRT ASP SFP
(The biscuits have been made.)

[19] *啲餅整好晒喇。*
di1 beng2 zing2 hou2 saai3 laa3
CL biscuit make PRT PRT SFP
(The biscuits are all made.)

Adverbs

Adverbs may modify verbs, adjectives and sentences. Adverbial modification of verbs and/or adjectives can be done using one of these three means: 1) the use of the adverbial marker *得 dak1* + adjective as in [20], 2) reduplication of adjectives with or without the suffix *地 dei2* as in [21] and 3) the use of adjective + *咁 gam2* + verb as in [22]. The first adverbial modifier appears after the verb, and the other two appear before the verb or the adjective.

[20] *你食得好快喎！*
nei5 sik6 dak1 hou2 faai3 wo3
you eat ADV very fast SFP
(You eat very fast!)

[21] *你乖乖地食飯先。*
nei5 gwaai1-gwaai1-dei2 sik6 faan6 sin1
you well-behaved-well-behaved+PRT eat rice first
(You behave and eat first.)

[22] *你細細聲咁講俾我聽啦。*
nei5 sai3-sai3-seng1 gam2 gong2 bei2 ngo5 teng1 laa1
you small-small-sound thus tell to I hear SFP
(Tell me in a very soft voice.)

There are two types of sentence adverbs. Temporal adverbs (e.g., *都 dou1* [also]), adverbs of scope (e.g., *仲 zung6* [still]) and reduplicated time words for indicating frequency (e.g., *日日 jat6jat6* 'day-day' [every day]), must appear immediately before the verb as in [23]. Other sentence adverbs (e.g., *差啲 caa1di1* [almost]) may appear immediately before the verb or at the beginning of the sentence as in [24].

[23] *我三樣都要。*
ngo5 saam1 joeng6 dou1 jiu3
I three CL also want
(I want all three of them.)

[24] *差啲佢就攞金牌 喇！*
caa1di1 keoi5 zau6 lo2 gam1 paai4 gaa3 laa3
almost s/he then take gold medal SFP SFP
(S/he almost got the gold medal!)

Prepositions

In Chinese, prepositions (e.g., *喺 hai2* [at], *同 tung4* [with]) express the relation between the two noun phrases. In some ways, prepositions function like verbs. Some prepositions may occur in a sentence on their own without a verb as in [25]. Some may take aspect markers as in [26], verbal particles as in [27], form A-not-A questions as in [28] and be modified by reduplicated adjectives as in [29].

[25] *細佬喺屋企。*
sai3lou2 hai2 uk1kei2
younger-brother PREP home
(The younger brother is at home.)

[26] *我同緊細佬玩。*
ngo5 tung4 gan2 sai3lou2 waan2
I PREP ASP younger-brother play
(I am playing with my younger brother.)

[27] *啲玩具喺晒屋企。*
di1 wun6geoi6 hai2 saai3 uk1kei2
CL toy PREP PRT home
(The toys are all at home.)

[28] *媽咪喺唔喺屋企啊？*
maa1mi4 hai2-m4-hai2. uk1kei2 aa3
mommy PREP-not-PREP home SFP
(Is Mommy at home?)

[29] *你靜靜地喺房度啦。*
nei5 zing6-zing2-dei2 hai2. fong2 dou6 laa1
you quiet-quiet+PRT PREP room PRT SFP
(You stay in the room quietly.)

Postpositions or localizers

Localizers, or postpositions, are expressions of location that often end with the morpheme *邊 bin6* or *面 min6* (e.g., *上邊 soeng6bin6* 'up-side' [above], *入面 jap-6min6* 'in-side' [inside]). These expressions can immediately follow a preposition as in [30] or a prepositional phrase as in [31].

[30] *架車喺上邊。*
gaa3 ce1 hai2 soeng6bin6
CL car PREP above
(The car is up there.)

[31] *喺個盒入面*
hai2. go3 hap2 jap6min6
PREP CL box inside
(Inside the box.)

Conjunctions

In Cantonese, while phrases can be put together explicitly with the conjunction 同埋 *tung4maai4* [and] or 同 *tung4* [and] as in [32], they are often juxtaposed without explicit markings as in [33]. Similarly, while clauses can be conjoined by a single conjunction or a pair of conjunctions, it is also common to have two clauses juxtaposed. In the latter case, the logical relations between the clauses must be inferred from the discourse and broader communication context. The use of conjunctions in clauses is further discussed and illustrated in Section 1.8.

[32] *等我買啲蘋果同橙先啦。*
dang2 ngo5 maai5 di1 ping4gwo2 tung4 caang2 sin1 laa1
let I buy CL apple CONJ orange first SFP
(Let me buy some apples and oranges first.)

[33] *等我幫你買啲衫褲鞋襪先啦。*
dang2 ngo5 bong1 nei5 maai5 di1 saam1 fu3 haai4 mat6 sin1 laa1
let I help you buy CL shirt pants shoe sock first SFP
(Let me help you buy some shirts, pants, shoes and socks first.)

Sentence final particles, topic particles and clause-final particles

Sentence final particles (e.g., *㗎 gaa3*, *喇 laa3*, *囉 lo1*) appear primarily at the end of a sentence. Their functions are to indicate speech act types (e.g., questions as in [34], assertions as in [35] and requests), mark evidentiality or add affective and emotional nuances to the speaker's proposition (Matthews & Yip, 2011). In some sentences, final particles can occur in combinations to add subtle affective nuances to the speaker's message as in [36]. With about 30 in number, sentence final particles are a characteristic feature of Cantonese.

[34] *媽咪呢？*
maa1mi4 le1
mommy SFP
(Where is Mommy?)

[35] *係喇！*
hai6 laa3
be SFP
(Yes!)

[36] *你仲食？你已經食咗三個喇喎！*
nei5 zung6 sik6? nei5 ji5ging1 sik6 zo2 saam1 go3 laa3 wo3
you still eat? you already eat ASP three CL SFP SFP
(You are still eating? You have already eaten three of these!)

Some particles (e.g., *呀 aa4* and *呢 le1*) occur after the topic in order to draw attention to it. Oftentimes, a pause follows the topic particle as in [37]. Some particles (e.g., *喎 wo3*, *喇 laa3*) occur at the end of a clause, as in [38], drawing attention to the clause that follows.

[37] *媽咪呢，最鍾意食士多啤梨蛋糕 喇。*
maa1mi4 le1, zeoi3 zung1ji3 sik6 si6do1be1lei2 daan6gou1 gaa3 laa3
mommy PRT, most like-to eat strawberry cake SFP SFP
(Mommy likes strawberry cakes the most.)

[38] *你聽清楚喎，三點鐘等呀。*
nei5 teng1 cing1co2 wo3, saam1 dim2zung1 dang2 aa3
you listen clearly PRT, three o'clock wait SFP
(Listen carefully; (we) wait for each other at three o'clock.)

Interjections and onomatopoeia

Interjections are words or sounds (e.g., *呀 aa3*, *哩 le1*) that are meaningless to the message being conveyed as illustrated in [39]. Sometimes, they fill a pause or transition between sentences and clauses. Onomatopoeic expressions are often formed by reduplication of syllables that end with the noun 聲 *seng1* [sound] to mimic certain sounds as in [40].

[39] *e6，咁你就三點哩先嚟啦。*
e6, gam2 nei5 zau6 saam1 dim2 le1 sin1 lei4 laa1
INT, so you then three o'clock INT first come SFP
(Umm, so then you can come at three o'clock.)

[40] *佢瞓到咯咯聲。*
keoi5 fan3 dou3 gok4gok4-seng1
s/he sleep to-the-extent ONO-sound
(S/he is really sound asleep.)

1.4 Phrases and their different types

A phrase contains one or more words that are put together according to a set of rules, with one of the words serving as its head. The head determines the syntactic status of the entire phrase. For example, a verb phrase like [41] has a verb as its head. In addition to verbs, nouns, adjectives and prepositions can also serve as the heads of phrases. [42], [43] and [44] give examples of a noun phrase, an adjectival phrase and a prepositional phrase, respectively.

[41] *整好咗*
zing2 hou2 zo2
make finish ASP
(made (it))

[42] *三個糉*
saam1 go3 zung2
three CL rice-dumpling
(three rice dumplings)

[43] *好開心*
hou2 hoi1sam1
very happy
(very happy)

[44] *喺枱度*
hai2 toi2 dou6
at table PRT
(at the table)

1.5 Clauses and sentences

A sentence is formed when words and phrases are put together in a proper order according to some syntactic principles. In a Cantonese sentence, the two main structural constituents are 1) a clause or several clauses, and/or 2) one or two sentence final particles. A clause can assume the status of a sentence when it conveys a proposition and, most importantly, when it is not contained in another clause. [45] is a clause as well as a sentence. A clause conveys a proposition that is generally expressed in the form of subject-predicate.

[45] *呢架車係我！*
nei1 gaa3 ce1 hai6 ngo5 gaa3
this CL car be I POSS
(This car is mine!)

As Fung (2009) pointed out, defining clauses and sentences in Chinese is far from straightforward. In many Indo-European languages, a full sentence typically includes a subject that is filled by a noun phrase and a predicate that is filled by a finite verb. In Chinese, there are many subject-predicate sentences of this kind, but there are no finiteness markings on the verb as in [46]. In Cantonese, the subject does not have to be a noun phrase; it can be an adjective as in [47], a verb phrase as in [48] or left unexpressed as in [49]. In addition, the predicate in a Cantonese sentence does not have to be a verb; it can be an adjective as in [50] or another noun as in [51], appearing right after the subject without a linking verb.

[46] *媽咪炒緊餸。*
maa1mi4 caau2 gan2 sung3
mommy stir-fry ASP dishes
(Mommy is stir-frying vegetables/meat.)

[47] *誠實最緊要。*
sing4sat6 zeoi3 gan2jiu3
honest most important
(Being honest is the most important thing.)

[48] *飲多啲水最緊要。*
jam2 do1 di1 seoi2 zeoi3 gan2jiu3
drink more a-bit water most important
(Drinking more water is the most important thing to do.)

[49] *落雨喇！*
lok6 jyu5 laa3
fall rain SFP
((It's) raining!)

[50] *黃小姐好靚。*
wong4 siu2ze2 hou2 leng3
Wong Miss very pretty
(Miss Wong is very pretty.)

[51] *今日假期呀。*
gam1jat6 gaa3kei4 aa3
today holiday SFP
(Today is a holiday.)

1.6 Canonical and non-canonical word order

The canonical word order in Chinese sentences is subject-verb-object (SVO), like many subject-predicate languages. The initial position in a sentence can be taken up by the thematic role of the agent – that is, the person who performs the action encoded by the verb – as in [52], but it does not always. In fact, the patient-object can be moved to the front of the sentence as in [53] in a process called topicalization.

[52] *姐姐做緊功課。*
ze4ze1 zou6 gan2 gung1fo3
older-sister do ASP homework
(The older sister is doing homework.)

[53] *個碟我擺咗上去枱度喇。*
go3 dip2 ngoi5 baai2 zo2 soeng5 heoi3 toi2 dou6 laa3
CL plate I put ASP up go table PRT SFP
(I have put the plate on the table.)

Postposing the subject, also known as right dislocation, is another change to the canonical word order of a sentence that is often seen in conversational speech. In [54], the speaker puts the subject of the sentence back in as an afterthought, and this can happen when the speaker rushes to give the new information first.

[54] *去咗買餸喇，媽咪。*
heoi3 zo2 maai5 sung3 laa3 maa1mi4
go ASP buy grocery SFP mother
(Mom has gone grocery shopping.)

Passive sentences do not follow the canonical word order. Compare the active sentence [55] and the passive sentence [56]. In passives, the argument representing the patient takes up the role of the grammatical subject in [56], which then precedes the argument representing the agent. The agent is introduced by the prepositional *俾 bei2* [by] phrase. In Cantonese, the noun phrase following the *俾 bei2* [by] cannot be omitted. Passive sentences are less common in Cantonese than in English. There are at least two reasons for this. Passive sentences are often used when the action affects the patient in an adverse manner. Instead of passivization, the patient can be moved to the beginning of the sentence through topicalization, as in [57].

[55] *個女仔踢咗婆婆一腳。*
go3 neoi5zai2 tek3 zo2 po4po2 jat1 goek3
CL girl kick ASP old-lady one foot
(The girl has given the old lady a kick.)

[56] *個婆婆俾個女仔踢咗一腳。*
go3 po4po2 bei2 go3 neoi5zai2 tek3 zo2 jat1 goek3
CL old-lady by CL girl kick ASP one foot
(The old lady has been given a kick by the girl.)

[57] *架車整好咗喇。*
gaa1 ce1 zing2 hou2 zo2 laa3
CL car fix finish ASP SFP
(The car has been fixed.)

In addition to subject, topic is another grammatical notion in Chinese sentences. In fact, sentence topic plays a key role in Chinese grammar. A sentence topic has three properties. First, it appears in the initial position of a sentence. Second, it "specifies the time, place, or circumstances to which the rest of the sentence applies" (Matthews & Yip, 2011, p. 84) and comments on. Third, as can be inferred from the second property, the sentence topic does not always have a grammatical relation to the predicate. In [58], the topic place is not the subject of any action but indicates the place to which the predicate – that is, growing flowers – applies.

[58] *呢個地方，最適合種花。*
nei1 go3 dei6fong1, zeoi3 sik1hap6 zung3 faa1
this CL place, most suitable grow flower
(This place is most suited for growing flowers.)

1.7 Sentence types according to internal structures

According to their internal structure, sentences can be classified either as simple, complex or compound (Zhan & Bai, 2016). A simple sentence [59] has only one clause. A complex sentence [60] has a main clause and one or more subordinate clauses embedded within it. A compound sentence [61] consists of two or more clauses, and the clauses are not embedded within each other.

[59] *爸爸去咗打波。*
baa4baa1 heoi3 zo2 daa2 bo1
daddy go ASP play ball
(Daddy has gone to play ball.)

[60] *佢聽到有人敲門。*
keoi5 teng1 dou2 jau5 jan4 haau1 mun4
s/he hear PRT have person knock door
(S/he heard someone knocking on the door.)

[61] *姐姐要煮飯，同埋洗衫。*
ze4ze1 jiu3 zyu2 faan6, tung4maai4 sai2 saam1
older-sister need-to cook rice and wash clothes
(The older sister needs to cook and do the laundry.)

In Chinese, it is not easy to make a distinction between compound and complex sentences. One reason is that the subordinate and dependent clause in a complex sentence may not necessarily be embedded within or contained inside the main clause, but rather, occurs outside it (Zhan & Bai, 2016). [62] illustrates a complex sentence with the subordinate clause introduced by a pause and the causal conjunction 所以 *so2ji5* [so]. Such a subordinate clause looks like part of a compound sentence that contains coordinated clauses. Compare [62] and the compound sentence [63] formed by the coordinating conjunction *或者waakze2* [or]. Note that in Chinese, there is an absence of formal finiteness markings on the verbs or other linguistic devices that make a distinction between subordinate clauses and coordinated clauses.

[62] *你今日嚟咗，所以我聽日就唔使去喇。*
nei5 gam1jat6 lei4 zo2, so2ji5 ngo5 ting1jat6 zau6 m4sai2 heoi3 laa3
you today come ASP, so I tomorrow then no-need-to go SFP
(Because you have come today, so I don't have to go tomorrow.)

[63] *你今日拎嚟呢度，或者聽日俾佢都得呀。*
nei5 gam1jat6 ling1 lei4 nei1dou6, waak6ze2 ting1jat6 bei2 keoi5 dou1 dak1 aa3
you today bring come here, or tomorrow give s/he also can SFP
(You can bring (it) here today, or (you) can give (it) to him/her tomorrow.)

Even if compound and complex sentences are collapsed into one single category of complex sentences to include all sentences containing more than one clause, identifying a complex sentence in Chinese as such can still be elusive. In sentences in which the subordinate clause is embedded within the main clause, there is no formal distinction of the verbs or word order changes that would mark it as a subordinate embedded clause (Zhan & Bai, 2016). In [64] the subject of the sentence *佢成日打機 keoi5 sing4jat6 daa2 gei1* [s/he plays computer games all day] is a clause in and of itself, which can appear independently as a sentence on its own in another context without any changes in form.

[64] *佢成日打機好唔聽話。*
keoi5 sing4jat6 daa2gei1 hou2 m4 teng1waa6
s/he all-day hit-machine (play electronic games) very not compliant
(S/he is not compliant and plays computer games all day.)

In Cantonese, serial verb constructions are important and very productive (Matthews, 2006). They express a range of meanings, including benefactive (as in [65]), directional (as in [66]), instrumental (as in [67]), purposive (as in [68] and [69]) and many others. In English, these same meanings are often expressed with the use of prepositions, as can be seen from the translation given in [67]. As is clear from the examples, serial verb constructions are a series of verbs that follow one another within the clause, without the presence of a conjunction between them or changes in form. The conventional definition of simple sentences does not credit the complexity involved in the conjugation of verbs within a single clause in serial verb constructions.

[65] *我幫你整番架車喇。*
ngo5 bong1 nei5 zing2 faan1 gaa3 ce1 laa3
I help you make back CL car SFP
(I helped you fix the car.)

[66] *弟弟拎咗個波出去。*
dai4dai2 ling1 zo2 go3 bo1 ceot1 heoi3
younger-brother take ASP CL ball out go
(The younger brother has taken the ball and gone out.)

[67] *媽咪用匙羹搞啲啫喱。*
maa1mi4 jung6 ci4gang1 gaau2 di1 ze1lei2
mommy use spoon stir CL jelly
(Mommy stirs the jelly with a spoon.)

[68] *我想去游水。*
ngo5 soeng2 heoi3 jau4seoi2
I want-to go swim
(I want to go swimming.)

[69] *我想去公園玩。*
ngo5 soeng2 heoi3 gung1jyun2 waan2
I want-to go park play
(I want to go play in the park.)

1.8 Logical relations between clauses

A complex sentence contains a main clause and one or more clauses. Conjunctions are often used to mark logical relations between clauses, including coordinating, temporal, concessive, conditional, causative and purposive relations. There are individual conjunctions (e.g., 或者 *waak6ze2* [or] as in [70]), as well as conjunction pairs (e.g., 雖然 . . . 但係 . . . *seoi1jin4 . . . daan6hai6 . . .* 'although . . . but . . . ' [although . . .]), (e.g., 無論 . . . 都 . . . *mou4leon6 . . . dou1 . . .* [no matter . . . still/also . . .]). [71] and [72] give examples of two different conjunction pairs.

[70] *你今日拎嚟呢度，或者聽日俾佢都得呀。*
nei5 gam1jat6 ling1 lei4 nei1dou6, waak6ze2 ting1jat6 bei2 keoi5 dou1 dak1 aa3
you today bring come here, or tomorrow give s/he also can SFP
(You bring (it) here today, or giving (it) to him/her tomorrow is also okay.)

[71] *隻公仔雖然好靚，但係太貴喇。*
zek3 gung1zai2 seoi1jin4 hou2 leng3, daan6hai6 taai3 gwai3 laa3
CL doll although very pretty, but too expensive SFP
(Although the doll is very pretty, (it) is too expensive.)

[72] *無論佢幾跩，媽咪都唔嬲佢。*
mou4leon6 keoi5 gei2 jai5, maa1mi4 dou1 m4 lau1 keoi5
no-matter s/he how naughty, mommy also not angry her
(No matter how naughty s/he is, Mommy does not get angry with him/her.)

In Chinese, it is not uncommon for two clauses to be juxtaposed in a sentence as in [73] and [74]. Without the explicit marking of the logical relation between the clauses, the meaning of the sentence has to be inferred from the discourse and broader communication context, occasionally resulting in ambiguous interpretations. [75] can have two interpretations, as can be seen in the English translations.

[73] *落雨，我哋唔去行山喇。*
lok6 jyu5, ngo5dei6 m4 heoi3 haang4 saan1 laa3
fall rain, we not go walk mountain SFP
(Because (it) is raining, we are not going hiking.)

[74] *你唔快啲嚟，我就食晒啲餅㗎喇。*
nei5 m4 faai3 di1 lei4, ngo5 zau6 sik6 saai3 di1 beng2 gaa3 laa3
you not fast a-bit come, I then eat all CL biscuit SFP SFP
((If) you don't come quickly, I will eat up the biscuits.)

[75] *你唔嚟，我就唔食。*
nei5 m4 lei4 ngo5 zau6 m4 sik6
you not come I then not eat
(If you do not come, then I won't eat.)
(Because you did not come, therefore I did not eat.)

In sentences with more than one clause, the clauses can be said to express conjunctive or disjunctive relations. In conjunctive sentences [76], both clauses have the same truth value and indicate temporal sequences or correlations. In disjunctive sentences [77], only one of the clauses is true, and the two clauses often represent two options or contradictory statements.

[76] *我踢完波，跟住去沖涼。*
ngo5 tek3 jyun4 bo1, gan1zyu6 heoi3 cung1loeng4
I kick finish ball, and-then go take-a-shower
(I finished playing football, and then I went to take a shower.)

[77] *你可以揀：一係去做功課，一係去瞓覺。*
nei5 ho2ji5 gaan2: jat1hai6 heoi3 zou6 gung1fo3, jat1hai6 heoi3 fan3gaau3
you may choose: either go do homework, either go sleep
(You may choose: either go and do your homework, or go to sleep.)

1.9 Sentence types according to communicative functions

According to communicative functions, there are four sentence types: declaratives, interrogatives, exclamatives and imperatives. In this section, we focus on the key features of interrogatives, exclamatives and imperatives in Chinese.

First of all, no changes in the canonical word order of declarative sentences are required in the formation of interrogatives. In other words, the *wh*-word in Chinese questions remain in situ as in [78]. There are six major types of questions in Cantonese: 1) yes/no questions, 2) alternative questions, 3) *wh* questions, 4) indirect questions, 5) multiple questions and 6) exclamatory questions. The different types of yes/no questions and *wh* questions are described in detail in Chapter 2 on the *Grammatical Analysis of Cantonese Samples* (GACS) framework.

Alternative questions (as in [79]) are choice questions, in which two alternatives are provided with the conjunction *定係 ding6hai6* [or], or *定 ding6* [or] for short, in between. Indirect questions (as in [80]) are formed by simply adding a verb of report directly before the direct questions. Cantonese questions may ask for two or more pieces of information, and these multiple questions are often asked indirectly as in [81]. Exclamatory questions (as in [82]) do not expect an answer and often sound rhetorical.

[78] *婆婆最錫邊個？*
po4po2 zeoi3 sek3 bin1go3
grandmother most like who
(Who does Grandmother like most?)

[79] *你想食橙定蘋果？*
nei5 soeng2 sik6 caang2 ding6 ping4gwo2
you want-to eat orange or apple
(Do you want to eat an orange or an apple?)

[80] *媽咪問你食乜嘢。*
maa1mi4 man6 nei5 sik6 mat1je5
mommy ask you eat what
(Mommy is asking you what you eat.)

[81] *你問我想幾時食乜嘢話？*
nei5 man6 ngo5 soeng2 gei2si4 sik6 mat1je5 waa2
you ask I want-to when eat what SFP
(What and when was that that you asked about whether I wanted to eat?)

[82] *咁點算呀？*
gam2 dim2syun3 aa3
so what-now SFP
(So what do (we) do?)

Exclamations can appear in statements and questions. Forms like *哎吔 ai1jaa1* [oops], *嘩 waa3* [whoa] and *咦 ji2* [huh] are used to express shock or disapproval, surprise or wonder, and surprise, respectively. [83] illustrates the use of *咦 ji2* to express surprise. Exclamatory questions with the words *點知 dim2zi1* [how do you know] or *唔通 m4tung1* [as if], like [84], behave like rhetorical questions to which an answer is not expected.

[83] *咦，我以為你唔嚟添。*
ji2, ngo5 ji5wai4 nei5 m4 lei4 tim1
INT, I think you not come SFP
(Huh, I thought you were not coming.)

[84] *唔通爸爸會鬧你咩！*
m4tung1 baa4baa1 wui5 naau6 nei5 me1
as-if daddy will scold you SFP
(As if Daddy would scold you!)

Imperatives are used to give commands, directions and requests. A sentence final particle often appears at the end of imperative sentences to tone them down, or the word *唔該 m4goi1* [thank you] is used to make them sound more polite. Note that the subject pronoun *你 nei5* [you] is present in [85] while it can be dropped in other contexts. The word *等 dang2* [let] can be used in phrases like *等我 dang2 ngo5* [let me] or *等佢 dang2 keoi5* [let him/her] to form first-person or third-person imperative sentences like [86]. The adverb *不如 bat1jyu4* [rather] in the first or second person imperative makes a suggestion as in [87]. Imperative sentences can be made negative with the use of words like *唔好 m4hou2* 'not-good' [do not] or *咪 mai5* [do not], as in [88].

[85] *你拎張櫈出去出面啦。*
nei5 ling1 zoeng1 dang3 ceot1 heoi3 ceot1min6 laa1
you take CL chair out go outside SFP
(You take the chair outside, (please).)

[86] *等我拎張櫈出去出面啦。*
dang2 ngo5 ling1 zoeng1 dang3 ceot1 heoi3 ceot1min6 laa1
let I take CL chair out go outside SFP
(Let me take the chair outside.)

[87] *不如我哋去睇戲吖？*
bat1jyu4 ngo5dei6 heoi3 tai2 hei3 aa1
rather we go watch movie SPF
(Would you rather go watch a movie?)

[88] *唔好掂個煲呀！*
m4hou2 dim3 go3 bou1 aa3
do-not touch CL pot SFP
(Don't touch the pot!)

1.10 Summary

Cantonese is the second most influential spoken form of Chinese. Each Cantonese syllable is marked by one of the six tones, and the same syllable may carry different tones, each representing different morphemes. Cantonese can be described as an analytic language because there is barely any inflectional or derivational morphology for marking person, gender, case, number (except for pronouns), tense or mood. It does, however, have bound morphemes like aspect markers and verbal particles for verb phrase modification. As a topic-comment language, the sentence topic does not always have a grammatical relation to the predicate. Since the sentence subject can be unexpressed when it can be inferred from the discourse and pragmatic context, and the verbs are not marked for finiteness, it is not always clear whether a sentence should be considered complex or not. In addition, it is not uncommon to have two or more verbs stacked together, forming a serial verb construction without the presence of any linking conjunctions. Last but not least, unlike any other SVO languages, the relative clause in Cantonese appears before, instead of after, the head noun, like other noun modifying phrases. Now that we have a brief overview of Cantonese grammar, we are ready to see how children tackle this problem space over time!

2

GRAMMATICAL ANALYSIS OF CANTONESE SAMPLES

With C. C.-H. Cheung, J. M.-W. Lo and E. K.-H. Wan

2.1 Grammar and language sample analysis

Grammar typically refers to the set of abstract rules we use to add markers to words to express notions like number, tense and aspect (morphology) and to put words together into sentences (syntax) (Ambridge & Lieven, 2011). Young children who are learning language(s) in their ambient environment learn these rules implicitly and incidentally, over time, from everyday interactions with people around them. To examine the development of grammatical rules, researchers have analyzed cross-sectional and longitudinal samples of children's language during conversation or narrative tasks since the early days of child language studies (see Nippold, 2021 for a historic review).

Language sample analysis has been an important research method for the study of child language in Cantonese. Using conversational and narrative samples, research studies reported on Cantonese-speaking preschool children's development in a range of language domains, including semantics (e.g., Klee et al., 2004) and discourse referencing (To, 2006; Wong & Johnston, 2004). In the domain of grammar, many studies provided description of preschool children's development of individual parts, including aspect markers (Leung, 1995), classifiers (Szeto, 1996; Tse et al., 2007), dative constructions (Chan, 2003; Wong et al., 2010), focus adverbs (Lee, 1996), modal auxiliaries and sentence final particles (Lee et al., 1996), noun phrases (Wong, C. S.-P., 1996), negation markers (Tam & Stokes, 2001), serial verb constructions (Fung, 2011), *wh* questions (Cheung, 1996; Li et al., 2013; Wong & Ingram, 2003) and the polysemous form 俾bei2 (Wong, C. H., 1996; Wong, R. K.-S., 2004). Using summative measures obtained from narrative samples, two studies reported on language development in school-aged children. Wong et al. (2004) examined relative clauses, serial verb constructions, coordinate clauses, subordinate clauses, pre-transitive sentences and passive sentences.

DOI: 10.4324/9780367824013-2

To et al. (2010) examined vocabulary, complex syntax, character referencing and conjunctions. Their complex syntax measure included relative clauses, clausal complements, Manner Adverbs and preposition phrases.

2.2 Conversational samples in Cantonese

Most studies on preschool children's development of Cantonese grammar come from two conversational databases. They are the cross-sectional corpus from the International Educational Achievement Preschool Project (IEA Corpus) (Opper, 1996) and the longitudinal Hong Kong Cantonese Child Language Corpus (CANCORP) (Lee, Wong, C., Leung et al., 1996). In addition to these two, there are the relatively more recent cross-sectional conversational corpora: the University of Hong Kong 70X Corpus (HKU-70X) (Fletcher et al., 2000) and the Can-LARSP corpus (Leung & Li, 2016). Of the four databases, the CANCORP and the HKU 70X are publicly accessible through the CHILDES at https://childes.talkbank.org. Table 2.1 summarizes critical details of the four databases.

With a larger number of child participants, the three cross-sectional databases (Fletcher et al., 2000; Leung & Li, 2016; Opper, 1996) provided useful data for constructing a more comprehensive profile of how all the main components of Cantonese grammar develop in children over time during the preschool years. Tse (2006) and Tse and Li (2011) used the IEA corpus to "establish a normative framework of developmental milestones for children" (Tse & Li, 2011, p. 12) three, four and five years. Fletcher et al. (2000) drew up a profile of language development in two-, three-, four- and five-year-old children using the CANCORP and the HKU-70X corpus. Leung and Li (2016) used the Can-LARSP corpus to develop a comprehensive grammatical analysis framework for the assessment of language in children between two and six years of age. These profiles provide a useful reference for early childhood educators for curriculum planning and for speech-language therapists for screening for and diagnosis of language disorder and for intervention planning.

2.3 The *Grammatical Analysis of Cantonese Samples* (GACS) framework: key features

In this book, we build on lessons from the earlier studies and use a new framework of grammatical analysis to profile the development of Cantonese in typically developing preschool children and to describe the language problems observed in children with developmental language disorder. In this chapter, our focus is on the framework.

The *Grammatical Analysis of Cantonese Samples* (GACS) framework is designed for clinical use by speech-language therapists and child language researchers to conduct comprehensive analyses of children's grammar using conversational samples. GACS has three new features, and we will describe each of these features one by one.

TABLE 2.1 Critical details of the four databases on Cantonese grammar development

	IEA corpus	*CANCORP*	*HKU-70X*	*Can-LARSP corpus*
Date	1996	1996	2000	2016
Age of children	3;–5;11	Start age: 1;5–2;0 End age: 2;7–3;8	2;5–5;8	2;1–5;11
No. of children	164	8	70	119
Sampling of children	68 preschools in different parts of Hong Kong	Personal contacts	1 kindergarten	6 kindergartens and 4 nurseries
No. of groups	3 age groups with 82 boys and 82 girls each	Nil	7 age groups with 5 boys and 5 girls each	6 age groups with 5 to 24 children in each group
Sampling frame	Once	Bi-weekly for about a year, resulting in 19 to 27 samples per child	Once	Once
No. of utterances per child	About 50 per on average	Variable, typically over 100	100	50
Communication partner	Same-aged peer	Family member(s) and trained research assistants	Trained research assistants	Trained research assistants
Activities	Play with a standard set of toys	Spontaneous play	Play with a standard set of toys	Free play with toys
Location	Kindergarten	Home	Kindergarten	Unknown
Key reference	Tse (2006) Tse and Li (2011)	Lee et al. (1996)	Fletcher et al. (2000)	Leung and Li (2016)

A different theoretical basis

Instead of taking a theoretical approach of adult grammar as in Leung and Li (2016), we developed the GACS framework on the basis of functionalist, or usage-based, constructivist theories of language development (e.g., Bates & MacWhinney, 1982; Bates et al., 1991; Goldberg, 2006; Tomasello, 2003). One key assumption of these theories is that communication drives language development. Communication involves transfer of information and the development and maintenance of social relationships. The ultimate goal for a child is to develop culturally appropriate social-interaction skills and linguistic knowledge to engage in effective and efficient communication with people in his/her community.

To become effective speakers, children need to be optimally informative in their utterances. When talking about people, objects and events, children need to include details such as quantity, color, size and location for their listeners to readily identify who or what they refer to with minimal effort. That provides the motivation for children to learn how to expand their noun phrases using adjectives, relative clauses or other modifiers. When talking about actions and movements, children need to provide details such as possibility, temporal contour, result, direction, manner and path for their listeners to readily identify the perspective they have chosen to take. That provides the motivation for children to learn how to expand their verb phrases using modal auxiliaries, particles, adverbs or other modifiers.

To become effective speakers, children also need to make appropriate use of the linguistic options available to them at two levels. First, they need to use the most suitable sentence type to achieve the communicative function intended. That provides the motivation for children to learn how to use imperative sentences to give commands and regulate others' behaviors; declarative sentences to make comments about people, objects and events; and interrogative sentences to find out different information about people and the world. Second, they need to use the most suitable construction to communicate to the listeners their chosen perspective on the event. That provides the motivation for children to expand their repertoire of syntactic constructions from canonical sentences to sentences following non-canonical word order such as passive sentences and topicalized sentences.

As they grow, children develop complex thoughts involving causes, predictions, intention and time. Speaking is a temporal event; hence, a speaker is under pressure to effectively and efficiently encode an optimal amount of complex information in a sentence for successful processing by his/her listeners. To become efficient speakers, children need to learn how to package a linearly ordered chain of events into hierarchically organized clauses to form sentences and a coherent discourse (Berman & Slobin, 1994). That provides the motivation for children to learn how to put clauses together, embed one clause in another to form complex sentences, use different conjunctions to indicate temporal and logical relationships and use cohesive devices appropriately in discourse.

Language development is a process in which children learn the skills and knowledge to overcome the physical, cognitive and psychosocial challenges in oral communication in real time. It is the pressure in meeting these challenges that motivates children to learn all the complex as well as the nuanced aspects of grammar in order to become members of their language community. Building on functionalist or usage-based constructivist theories of language development, the GACS framework directs speech-language therapists' attention to children's use of grammar in the service of communicative functions (Bates et al., 1991) during assessment and intervention.

A type-based scoring system

Following the example of the Index of Productive Syntax (Scarborough, 1990), the GACS uses a type-based scoring system, in which four unique exemplars for each included item are identified and scored. For example, for an item like Classifiers, speech-language therapists will look for a maximum of four different Classifiers in the child's conversational sample. Hence, the same classifier (e.g., *個 go3*) and, in the same fashion, the same Aspect Marker (e.g., *咗 zo2*) or the same Sentence Final Particle (e.g., *喇 laa3*) is scored only once. Four is a considered a good number to ascertain if a child has some abstract knowledge of the item. The items include grammatical forms (e.g., Classifiers, Aspect Markers), clauses (e.g., Relative Clauses, Clauses with Conjunctions, Clausal Complements) and larger-size units (e.g., Subject-Verb-Object structures, Serial Verb Constructions, Sentences with a Prepositional Phrase).

A clear definition of the items

Unlike the earlier studies (Fletcher et al., 2000; Leung & Li, 2016; Tse & Li, 2011), the GACS framework provides a clear linguistic definition of each of the items, with examples that allow speech-language therapists to complete an objective and systematic analysis of a child's grammar that can then be replicated by others. The definitions are largely based on the seminal works on Cantonese grammar by Cheung (2007) and Matthews and Yip (2011). They are given in the remainder of this chapter. Items in the framework were selected following our thorough review of the literature on language development on the basis of our clinical experience as speech-language therapists and our linguistic intuition as native speakers of Cantonese.

2.4 The GACS framework: an overview

The GACS framework is designed for use with children with a range of language abilities, from those who put two to three words together to those who use sentences. It is best used for the analysis of conversational samples. While it is not a requirement of the framework per se, a useful analysis will result from a sample that is representative of the child's actual language ability. A sample of at least 50 utterances is recommended.

The items in the framework are grouped into five sections: Noun Phrase Expansion, Verb Phrase Expansion, Sentence Structures, Questions, and last but not least, Sentence Adverbs, Conjunctions and Sentence Final Particles. The organization of items into Noun Phrase Expansion, Verb Phrase Expansion, Sentence Structures and Questions sections in the GACS framework is not new. It has been used previously in systematic analysis (Miller, 1981; Scarborough, 1990) and description (Fletcher & O'Toole, 2016) of language development in English-speaking children for clinical purposes. In the GACS, items within the sections are ordered somewhat developmentally based on our best knowledge from the literature on Cantonese, although much research is still needed to ascertain the order of emergence and mastery of various grammatical structures. Again, given the lack of developmental information for many of the grammatical structures, all exemplars are worth the same number of points. The total number of points for Noun Phrase Expansion is 28; for Verb Phrase Expansion is 56; for Sentence Structures is 100; for Questions is 40; and for Sentence Adverbs, Conjunctions and Sentence Final Particles is 48. The Grand Total is 272 points. Please refer to Wong et al. (2021a) for a copy of the summary score sheet for GACS.

Individual differences in children's language ability are well reported in the literature (Brown, 1973; Well, 1985). Given that the GACS framework is designed primarily for use by speech-language therapists and child language researchers working with children who are at risk for or who have language disorders, some of the more complex but less frequently observed forms and structures that are seen in linguistically advanced children (e.g., cleft sentences or right dislocation) are not included.

Given the absence of normative data on GACS scores that are collected from a representative and sizable sample of children, a child's score cannot be used for screening or diagnostic purposes. The scores, however, can be used to document the progress of individual children if the conversational samples used for the comparison are collected in a comparable manner and context. Before normative data on the GACS scores are available, the framework is best used for qualitative and descriptive purposes.

2.5 The GACS framework: notes on scoring

1. Before the analysis, cross out the fillers, mazes and self-corrections (e.g., *媽咪話,媽咪問我 . . . maa1mi4 waa6, maa1mi4 man6 ngo5 . . .* [Mom says, Mom asks me . . .]) and analyze the final version of the child's utterance. It is important, however, to write down the utterance in its original form with the fillers, mazes and self-corrections in the GACS summary sheet as frequent use of these speech interruptions can be indicative of sentence formulation problems.
2. Only credit forms and structures that are not an imitation of the adult utterance immediately before the child's utterances.
3. Credit is not given if the forms or structures do not map onto what actually was going on or what the child was intended to mean as far as it could be inferred from the context. In sentence [1], the context requires the child to use the modal *會 wui5* [will], indicating a future action, rather the Aspect Marker *咗 zo2*. The use of *咗 zo2* is hence considered inappropriate and is not given credit.

    [1] *呢道門撞咗人呀！*
    nei1 dou6 mun4 zong6 zo2 jan4 aa3
    this CL door knock-down ASP people SFP
    (This door has knocked people down!)

4. The same utterance (statements or questions) can receive credit in more than one section in the GACS. For sentence [2], the child receives three points: one in Section A Noun Phrase Expansion for *張櫈 zoeng1 dang3* [CL chair], one in Section B Verb Phrase Expansion *推番 teoi1 faan1* [push back] and one in Section C Sentence Structures (as directional Serial Verb Construction).

[2] *你推番張凳去前面。*
nei5 teoi1 faan1 zoeng1 dang3 heoi3 cin4min6
you push back CL chair go front
(You push the chair back to the front.)

5. Give the child credit if the sentence is generally well formed except for some minor errors in its non-core elements. For sentence [3], the child receives one point in Section C Sentence Structures for the benefactive serial verb construction despite a problem in word choice, using *綁 bong2* [tie] for *包紮 baau1zaat3* [wind a bandage around the wound].

[3] *幫佢綁傷口。*
bong1 keoi5 bong2 soeng1hau2
help he/she tie wound
((I) help him/her wind a bandage around the wound.)

6. Similarly, give the child credit in other sections, even if the child's sentence is ill formed and hence does not get a point in Section C Sentence Structures. For sentence [4], which could be an attempt to produce a passive sentence, the child receives a point in Section B Verb Phrase Expansion for *拎咗 ling1 zo2* [take ASP].

[4] *架飛機拎咗哥哥。*
go3 fei1gei1 ling1 zo2 go4go1
CL airplane take ASP big-brother
(The airplane has taken my big brother.)

7. For *wh* questions, the child's response must include other elements in addition to the *wh* word and/or the sentence final particle. For example, *邊度呀 bin1dou6 aa1?* [where PRT SFP] is not given credit. In contrast, the child is given credit if s/he produces an elaborated *where* question as in [5].

[5] *擺架車喺邊度呀？*
baai2 gaa3 ce1 hai2 bin1dou6 aa3
put CL car at where SFP
(Where do (we) put the car?)

8. In Section E Sentence Adverbs, Conjunctions and Sentence Final Particles, the child does not have to include the two main clauses or both the main and the embedded clauses to get credit. In conversation, especially in response to a question or a comment, often only one clause of the complex sentence is necessary. Sentence [6], with the use of an appropriate conjunction, is given credit under Causal Conjunctions.

[6] *因爲冇鬧鐘囉。*
jan1wai6 mou5 naau6zung1 lo1
because not-have alarm-clock SFP
(Because (I) don't have an alarm clock.)

9. Errors provide useful information on the child's zone of proximal development and, hence, on the selection of intervention goals. Error analysis is therefore the most important part of a language sample analysis. The five common types of errors include addition, omission, wrong choice of words, wrong order of words and sentence formulation. More than one error or error type can appear in a sentence. It is best for the speech-language therapist, the early childhood educator or the child language researcher who has collected the sample to complete the error analysis. The reason is that this person can make use of information from the linguistic, social and physical contexts of the conversation to assist his/her interpretation of the child's errors.

The GACS framework

A. Noun Phrase Expansion (NP) *名詞短語擴展*

1. Classifiers (Cl) *量詞*
2. Possessive constructions (Poss) *領屬結構*
3. Adjectival modifiers (Adj Mod) *形容詞修飾語*
4. Nominal modifiers (Nom Mod) *名詞修飾語*
5. Locative modifiers (Loc Mod) *處所修飾語*
6. Prepositional modifiers (Prep Mod) *介詞修飾語*
7. Relative clauses (RC) *關係從句*

B. Verb Phrase Expansion (VP) *動詞短語擴展*

1. Auxiliaries (Aux) *助動詞*
   - 1.1 Modal auxiliaries (Mod Aux) *情態助動詞*
   - 1.2 Other auxiliaries (Oth Aux) *其他助動詞*
2. Verbal adverbs (V Adv) *修飾動詞短語的副詞*
   - 2.1 Manner Adverbs (Man Adv) *情態副詞*
   - 2.2 Negation Adverbs (Neg Adv) *否定副詞*
   - 2.3 Degree Adverbs (Deg Adv) *程度副詞*
3. Aspect markers (Asp) *體貌詞尾*
4. Verbal particles (VPrt) *動詞助詞*
   - 4.1 Resultative particles (Res Prt) *結果助詞*
   - 4.2 Directional particles (Dir Prt) *方位助詞*
   - 4.3 Potential particles (Pot Prt) *能性助詞*
   - 4.4 Other verbal particles (Oth VPrt) *其他動詞助詞*
5. Complements (Comp) *補語*
   - 5.1 Descriptive complements (Des Comp) *描述補語*
   - 5.2 Complements of extent (Ext Comp) *程度補語*
   - 5.3 Complements of location (Loc Comp) *處所補語*
     - 5.3.1 Localizers (Loc) *方位詞*
     - 5.3.2 Prepositional phrases (PP) *介詞短語*

C. Sentence Structures (SS) *句子結構*

1. Verb-object structure (VO) *動-賓結構*
2. Subject-verb-object structure (SVO) *主-動-賓結構*
3. Subject-verb structure (SV) *主語-動詞謂語結構*

4. Subject-adjective structure (SA) *主語-形容詞謂語結構*
5. Subject-noun structure (SN) *主語-名詞謂語結構*
6. Topic structure (Top) *主題句*
7. Existential constructions (EC) *存在句*
8. Comparative constructions (Com C) *比較句*
   - 8.1 Comparison of adjectives (Com A) *形容詞的比較*
   - 8.2 Comparing quantities (Com Qua) *數量的比較*
9. Pivotal constructions (PC) *兼語結構*
10. Passive structure (Pass) *被動句*
11. *將 zoeng1* construction (ZC) *「將」字句*
12. Sentences with a prepositional phrase (S PP) *包含介詞短語的句子*
    - 12.1 *俾 bei2* construction *「俾」字句*
    - 12.2 *喺 hai2* construction *「喺」字句*
    - 12.3 *對 deoi3* construction *「對」字句*
    - 12.4 *同 tung4* construction *「同」字句*
    - 12.5 *到 dou3* construction *「到」字句*
13. Clausal complements (CC) *賓語從句*
14. Serial verb constructions (SVC) *連動結構*
    - 14.1 Serial verb constructions: Simple (SVC-1) *簡單連動結構*
      - I. Benefactive *施惠*
      - II. Comitative *伴隨*
      - III. Instrumental *工具性*
      - IV. Directional *方位*
      - V. Purpose *目的*
      - VI. Sequential *順序*
      - VII. Alternating *往復*
      - VIII. Circumstance *情境*
      - XI. Posture *姿態*
    - 14.2 Serial verb constructions: Complex (SVC-2) *複雜連動結構*
15. Complex sentences without overt conjunctions (CS-Conj) *無連詞複句*

D. Questions (Q) *疑問句*

1. Yes/No questions (YN) *是非問句*
   - 1.1 Particle questions (Prt Q) *助詞問句*
   - 1.2 A-not-A questions (A Q) *正反問句*
   - 1.3 Copula questions (Cop Q) *「係咪」問句*
   - 1.4 *未 mei6* questions (*未 mei6* Q) *「未」問句*
   - 1.5 Existential questions (Exi Q) *存在問句*
   - 1.6 Tag questions (Tag Q) *附加問句*
   - 1.7 Intonation questions (Int Q) *語調問句*
   - 1.8 Echo questions (Ech Q) *反問問句*
2. *Wh* questions (WhQ) *特指問句*
   - 2.1 *Wh*-words (Wh-1) *疑問代詞*
     - I. "What" questions *「乜嘢/咩」疑問句*
     - II. "Who" questions *「邊個」疑問句*
     - III. "Where" questions *「邊度/邊庶」疑問句*
     - IV. "Why" and reason questions *「做乜/做咩/做乜嘢/點解」疑問句*

2.2 *Wh* words (Wh-2) *疑問代詞*
  I. "Which" questions *「邊+名量詞」疑問句*
  II. "How many/much" questions *「幾多」疑問句*
  III. "When" and time questions *「幾時」疑問句*
  IV. "How" questions *「點樣/點」疑問句*

E. Sentence Adverbs, Conjunctions and Sentence Final Particles
修飾句子的副詞、連詞、句末助詞
1. Sentence adverbs (S Adv) *修飾句子的副詞*
   1.1 Scope adverbs (Sco Adv) *範圍副詞*
   1.2 Temporal adverbs (Tem Adv) *時間副詞*
   1.3 Frequency Adverbs (Fre Adv) *頻率副詞*
   1.4 Modal adverbs (Mod Adv) *語氣副詞*
2. Conjunctions (Conj) *連詞*
   2.1 Coordinating conjunctions (Coor Conj) *並列連詞*
   2.2 Causal conjunctions (Caus Conj) *因果連詞*
   2.3 Concession conjunctions (Conc Conj) *轉折連詞*
   2.4 Conditional conjunctions (Cond Conj) *條件連詞*
   2.5 Temporal conjunctions (Temp Conj) *時間連詞*
   2.6 Purpose conjunctions (Purp Conj) *目的連詞*
3. Sentence final particles (SFP) *句末助詞*

Section A

Noun phrase expansion (NP)

名詞短語擴展

Definition: A noun can be modified and expanded by a classifier, a numeral, a demonstrative, a possessor, a bare adjective, a noun, a localizer indicating location, a prepositional phrase or a relative clause.

1. Classifiers (Cl) 量詞

Definition: Classifiers immediately precede the noun. There are mainly two types of classifiers: measural classifiers and sortal classifiers (Matthews & Yip, 1994, 2011). Measural classifiers specify the quantity of the head noun (e.g., *磅 bong6* [pound], *斤 gan1* [catty], *啲 di1* (denoting plurality)) while sortal classifiers classify the head noun in terms of its intrinsic features such as shape (e.g., *張 zoeng1* denotes flat objects) (Matthews & Yip, 1994, 2011). Both types of classifiers can be preceded by a numeral such as *一 jat1* [one], and a demonstrative (*呢 nei1* [this] or *嗰 go2* [that]).

個 go3 is the most common classifier, and it is the first classifier observed in children before 30 months (Frank et al., 2017; Tardif et al., 2008). It can be used to classify a head noun denoting people as well as a head noun that does not call for a more specific classifier (e.g., an abstract noun).

Examples

一斤椰菜
jat1 <u>gan1</u> je4coi3
one CL cabbage
(one catty of cabbage)

啲小朋友
<u>di1</u> siu2pang4jau5
CL child
(the/some children)

呢三張櫈
nei1 saam1 <u>zoeng1</u> dang3
this three CL chair
(these three chairs)

一個女仔
jat1 <u>go3</u> neoi5zai2
one CL girl
(one girl)

一個機會
jat1 <u>go3</u> gei1wui6
one CL opportunity
(one opportunity)

2. Possessive constructions (Poss) 領屬結構

<u>Definition:</u> Possessive constructions involve a noun functioning as a possessor, followed by another noun (e.g., *朋友 pang4jau5* [friend]) or another noun phrase (e.g., *個朋友 go3 pang4jau5* 'Cl friend') serving as a possessum (Matthews & Yip, 1994, 2011). A linking particle *嘅 ge3* (similar to *'s* in English) or the appropriate classifier may go between the two nominals.

Examples

<u>媽咪嘅</u>朋友
<u>maa1mi4 ge3</u> pang4jau5
mommy POSS friend
(Mommy's friend(s))

<u>媽咪</u>個朋友
<u>maa1mi4</u> go3 pang4jau5
mommy CL friend
(Mommy's friend)

3. Adjectival modifiers (Adj Mod) 形容詞修飾語

Definition: An adjectival modifier refers to the adjective that precedes and modifies a noun (e.g., *屋 uk1* [house]) or a noun phrase (e.g., *嗰三個女仔 go2 saam1 go3 neoi5zai2* [those three girls]) (Cheung, 2007; Sio, 2006). The adjective may encode size, shape, color or other properties. A linking particle *嘅 ge3* may be present between the adjective and the following noun or noun phrase.

Examples

大屋
daai6 uk1
big house
((a) big house(s))

熱咖啡
jit6 gaa3fe1
hot coffee
(hot coffee)

好靚嗰三個女仔
hou2 leng3 go2 saam1 go3 neoi5zai2
very pretty that three CL girl
(those three very pretty girls)

黃色嘅蝴蝶
wong4sik1 ge3 wu4dip2
yellow PRT butterfly
((a) yellow butterfly(/ies))

4. Nominal modifier (Nom Mod) 名詞修飾語

Definition: Nominal modifiers refer to a noun (e.g., *舊年 gau6nin2* 'old-year' [last year]) or a noun phrase (e.g., *嗰個銀包 go2 go3 ngan4baau1* [that wallet]) that modifies the noun or noun phrase that it precedes. A linking particle *嘅 ge3* may appear between the nominal modifier and the following noun or noun phrase. Unlike possessive constructions, the nominal modifier and the following noun or noun phrase do not indicate a meaning of possession.

Examples

舊年嗰三件衫
gau6nin2 go2 saam1 gin6 saam1
old-year that three CL shirt
(those three shirts from last year)

嗰個銀包嘅顏色
go2 go3 ngan4baau1 ge3 ngaan4sik1
that CL wallet PRT color
(the color of that wallet)

5. Locative modifiers (Loc Mod) 處所修飾語

Definition: Locative modifiers refer to a localizer (e.g., 裡邊 *leoi5bin6* 'in-side' [inside], *呢度 nei1dou6* [here], *嗰度 go2dou6* [there]) or a noun followed by a localizer (e.g., 枱上面 *toi2 soeng6min6* 'table above' [on the table]) that serves to specify the location of the following head noun. Typically, a linking particle *嘅 ge3* or a [demonstrative + numeral + classifier] sequence appears between the locative modifier and the head noun.

Examples

裡邊嘅公仔
leoi5bin6 ge3 gung1zai2
inside PRT doll
(the doll(s) inside)

裡邊嗰三個公仔
leoi5bin6 go2 saam1 go3 gung1zai2
inside that three CL doll
(those three dolls inside)

枱上面嘅書
toi2 soeng6min6 ge3 syu1
table above PRT book
(the book(s) on the table)

枱上面嗰三本書
toi2 soeng6min6 go2 saam1 bun2 syu1
table above that three CL book
(those three books on the table)

6. Prepositional modifiers (Prep Mod) 介詞修飾語

Definition: Prepositional modifier refer to the prepositional phrase (e.g., *喺張枱度/上面 hai2 zoeng1 toi2 dou6/soeng6min6* [on the table]) that precedes the noun or noun phrase it modifies. A linking particle *嘅 ge3* may appear between the prepositional modifier and the following noun or noun phrase.

Examples

喺張枱度/上面嘅杯
hai2 zoeng1 toi2 dou6/soeng6min6 ge3 bui1
at CL table PRT/above PRT cup
(the cup(s) that is/are on the table)

喺張枱度/上面嗰三本書
hai2 zoeng1 toi2 dou6/soeng6min6 go2 saam1 bun2 syu1
at CL table PRT/above that three CL book
(those three books that are on the table)

7. Relative clauses (RC) 關係從句

Definition: A relative clause is a clause containing a verb phrase (e.g., 戴眼鏡 *daai3 ngaan5geng2* [wear glasses]). A linking particle *嘅 ge3* appears between the relative clause and the noun phrase, which may consist of a noun (e.g., *女仔 neoi5zai2* [girl]) only or a noun phrase (e.g., *啲三個女仔 go2 saam1 go3 neoi5zai2* [those three girls], 個女仔 *go3 neoi5zai2* [the girl]) (Cheung & Li, 2012; Sio, 2006; Matthews & Yip, 1994, 2011). Instead of *嘅 ge3*, an appropriate classifier can be used to link the relative clause and the noun or noun phrase.

Examples

戴眼鏡嘅女仔
daai3 ngaan5geng2 ge3 neoi5zai2
wear glasses PRT girl
(the girl(s) who wear(s) glasses)

戴眼鏡嘅啲三個女仔
daai3 ngaan5geng2 ge3 go2 saam1 go3 neoi5zai2
wear glasses PRT that three CL girl
(those three girls who wear glasses)

戴眼鏡個女仔
daai3 ngaan5geng2 go3 neoi5zai2
wear glasses CL girl
(the girl who wears glasses)

戴眼鏡啲三個女仔
daai3 ngaan5geng2 go2 saam1 go3 neoi5zai2
wear glasses that three CL girl
(those three girls who wear glasses)

Section B

Verb phrase expansion (VP)

動詞短語擴展

Definition: The meaning of a verb or verb phrase can be modified by an auxiliary, a verbal adverb, an aspect marker, a verbal particle or a complement. In addition to a verb or a verb phrase, verbal adverbs, verbal particles and complements can modify an adjective or an adjective phrase.

1. Auxiliaries (Aux) 助動詞

Definition: Auxiliaries are typically followed by a main verb, except when the verb can be inferred from the context. They cannot take aspect markers or verbal particles.

1.1. Modal auxiliaries (Mod Aux) 情態助動詞

Definition: Modal auxiliaries are used to express possibility, permission, ability, necessity, wishes, obligation and other related concepts. All modal auxiliaries appear before the main verb (Matthews & Yip, 1994, 2011). Modal auxiliaries in 1.1.1. are observed in children before 30 months (Lee et al., 1996; Wong, 1998), and those in 1.1.2. are common ones that appear after 30 months.

1.1.1. Modal auxiliaries I

I. *會 wui5* [will/would]
II. *可以 ho2ji5* [can/could, may/might]
III. *唔使 m4sai2* [no need to]

1.1.2. Modal auxiliaries II

I. *要 jiu3* [want to, need to]
II. *想 soeng2* [want to, wish to]
III. *唔准 m4zeon2* [not allowed to]
IV. *識 sik1* [know how to]
V. *鍾意 zung1ji3* [like to, love to]
VI. *應該 jing1goi1* [should, ought to]

Examples

你可以出院喇！
nei5 ho2ji5 ceot1jyun2 laa3
you can leave-hospital SFP
(You can be discharged from the hospital!)

我想睇書呀。
ngo5 soeng2 tai2 syu1 aa3
I want-to see book SFP
(I want to read a book.)

佢自己識返學㗎。
keoi5 zi6gei2 sik1 faan1hok6 gaa3
s/he self know-how-to go-to-school SFP
(S/he knows how to go to school by himself/herself.)

1.2 Other auxiliaries (Oth Aux) 其他助動詞

Definition: The words *有 jau5* [have] and *冇 mou5* [not have] can be used as auxiliaries before a verb. When the sentence refers to the past, they emphasize the truth value of the event depicted by the sentence. When the sentence refers to a present event, it gives rise to a habitual reading (Matthews & Yip, 1994, 2011).

Examples

我今日都有去公園㗎。
ngo5 gam1jat6 dou1 jau5 heoi3 gung1jyun2 gaa3
I today also have go park SFP
(I also went to the park today.)

我日日都有做運動㗎。
ngo5 jat6jat6 dou1 jau5 zou6 wan6dung6 gaa3
I every-day also have do exercise SFP
(I do do exercise every day.)

2. Verbal adverbs (V Adv) 修飾動詞短語的副詞

Definition: Verbal adverbs serve to modify the verb phrase or the adjective phrase, rather than the entire sentence. Typically, they appear before the verb phrase or the adjective phrase. Unlike sentence adverbs, verbal adverbs cannot appear before the subject. They include Manner Adverbs, Negation Adverbs and Degree Adverbs.

2.1 Manner Adverbs (Man Adv) 情態副詞

Definition: Manner Adverbs depict the manner in which an event is carried out. Some are derived forms, such as adjective + (*咁 gam2* [thus]) and reduplicated adjective/verb + (*哋 dei2*) (Matthews & Yip, 1994, 2011; Wong, 2002).

Examples

佢特登嚟睇你㗎。
keoi5 dak6dang1 lei4 tai2 nei5 gaa3
s/he especially come see you SFP
(S/he came especially to see you.)

佢好大力咁踢我。
keoi5 hou2 daai6lik6 gam2 tek3 ngo5
s/he very big-strength thus kick I
(S/he kicked me very hard.)

佢唔小心跌倒。
keoi5 m4 siu2sam1 dit3 dou2
s/he not careful fall PRT
(S/he carelessly fell.)

佢偷偷地走咗。
keoi5 tau1tau1-dei2 zau2 zo2
s/he sneaky-sneaky+PRT leave ASP
(S/he has left secretly.)

慢慢行，唔好跑呀。
maan6-maan2 hang4, m4hou2 paau2 aa3
slow-slow walk, do-not run SFP
(Walk slowly; don't run.)

2.2 Negation Adverbs (Neg Adv) 否定副詞

<u>Definition:</u> Negation Adverbs (e.g., *唔 m4* [not], *未 mei6* [not yet], *咪 mai5* [do not] and *冇 mou5* [not have]) negate the presence of a state depicted by an adjective phrase or an action depicted by a verb phrase (Cheung, 2007; Wong, 2002).

Examples

唔好食。
<u>m4</u> hou2sik6
not tasty
((It) is not tasty.)

佢冇洗手呀。
keoi5 <u>mou5</u> sai2 sau2 aa3
s/he not-have wash hand SFP
(S/he did not wash his/her hands.)

2.3 Degree Adverbs (Deg Adv) 程度副詞

<u>Definition:</u> Degree Adverbs (e.g., *幾 gei2* [quite], *太 taai3* [too], *好 hou2* [very], *最 zeoi3* [most], *咁 gam3* [this]/[so]) are used to mark the degree or extent of a state depicted by an adjective or a stative verb (Cheung, 2007; Wong, 2002).

Examples

今日天氣好熱。
gam1jat6 tin1hei3 <u>hou2</u> jit6
today weather very hot
(It's very hot today.)

我最鍾意食花生。
ngo5 <u>zeoi3</u> zung1ji3 sik6 faa1sang1
I most like-to eat peanut
(I like to eat peanuts the most.)

3. Aspect markers (Asp) 體貌詞尾

<u>Definition:</u> Aspect markers mark the viewpoint aspect of a situation (Matthews & Yip, 1994, 2011). For instance, the perfective marker *咗 zo2* indicates a completed event and usually implies past time reference. Unlike English, Cantonese does not have any morphological markers for tense. The aspect markers in 3.1 are observed in children before 30 months (Lee et al., 1996; Leung, 1995), and those in 3.2 appear after 30 months.

3.1 Asp I

I. Perfective marker *咗 zo2*
II. Imperfective markers 緊 *gan2, 喺度 hai2dou6, 住 zyu6*

3.2 Asp II

III. Experiential marker *過 gwo3*
IV. Habitual markers *開 hoi1, 慣 gwaan3*
V. Delimitative marker *吓 haa5*
VI. Inchoative marker *起(上)嚟 hei2(soeng3)lei4, 落去 lok6heoi3*

Examples

搬緊屋
bun1 gan2 uk1
move ASP house
(moving house)

靜啲，佢喺度畫畫。
zing6 di1, keoi5 hai2dou6 waak6 waa2
quiet a-bit, s/he ASP draw picture
(Keep quiet; s/he is drawing.)

幫我揸住個杯。
bong1 ngo5 zaa1 zyu6 go3 bui1
help I hold ASP CL cup
(Help me hold the cup.)

你去過330未呀？
nei5 heoi3 gwo3 330 mei6 aa3
you go ASP 330 not-yet SFP
(Have you ever been to 330?)

我去開嗰間餐廳冇開呀。
ngo5 heoi3 hoi1 go2 gaan1 caan1teng1 mou5 hoi1 aa3
I go ASP that CL restaurant not-have open SFP
(The restaurant I usually go to is not open.)

睇吓我。
tai2 haa5 ngo5
see ASP I
(Have a look at me.)

佢食食吓突然嘔起上嚟。
keoi5 sik6-sik6-haa5 dak6jin4 au2 hei2soeng3lei4
s/he eat-eat-ASP suddenly throw-up ASP
(S/he suddenly started throwing up while she was eating.)

4. Verbal particles (VPrt) 動詞助詞

Definition: Verbal particles are particles that follow the verb to indicate result, direction, possibility or other functions (full details follow).

4.1 Resultative particles (Res Prt) 結果助詞

Definition: Resultative particles are used with a transitive verb to denote results, and they form resultative compounds with the verb. Examples include *飽 baau2* [full up], *錯 co3* [wrong], *掂 dim6* [successfully completed], *定 ding6* (indicating to be ready), *到 dou2* [indicating ability], *到 dou3* [arrive at], *完 jyun4* [finish]/[to the end], *好 hou2* 'good' [finish], *剩 zing6* [remain], *爛 laan6* [broken], *明 ming4* [clear], *滿 mun5* [full], *成 seng4* [with success], *死 sei2* 'die' [to death], *勻 wan4* [thoroughly] and *壞 waai6* [bad]/[malfunction] (Matthews & Yip, 2011, p. 243; see also Matthews & Yip, 1994).

Examples

整爛咗佢間屋。
zing2 laan6 zo2 keoi5 gaan1 uk1
make broken ASP s/he CL house
((Somebody)) has broken his/her house.)

煮好咗飯喇。
zyu2 hou2 zo2 faan6 laa3
cook finish ASP rice SFP
((I) have finished cooking the rice.)

我做完功課喇。
ngo5 zou6 jyun4 gung1fo3 laa3
I do finish homework SFP
(I finished doing my homework.)

開(唔)到個盒呀。
hoi1 (m4) dou2 go3 hap2 aa3
Open (not) PRT CL box SFP
((I) can(not) open the box.)

返到學校未呀你？
faan1-dou3-hok6haau6 mei6 aa3 nei5?
go-to-school+arrive-at not-yet SFP you
(Have you arrived at the school yet?)

憎死你。
zang1 sei2 nei5
hate die you
((I) hate you very much.)

4.2 Directional particles (Dir Prt) 方位助詞

Definition: Directional particles appear after a verb, either transitive or intransitive, to basically denote direction. They can be categorized into simple and compound directional particles. Simple directional particles include *嚟 lei4* [come], *去 heoi3*

[go], *上 soeng5* [up], *落 lok6* [down], *開 hoi1* [away], *埋 maai4* [close], *出 ceot1* [out], *入 jap6* [in], *過 gwo3* [past]/[over], *起 hei2* [up], *到 dou3* [arrive at] and *番 faan1* [back] (Cheung, 2007, pp. 116–119). Note that in Matthews and Yip (2011), *到 dou3* [arrive at] is treated as a resultative particle.

Compound directional particles can be disyllabic or tri-syllabic. The disyllabic ones involve the combination of *上 soeng5* [up], *落 lok6* [down], *開 hoi1* [away], *埋 maai4* [close], *出 ceot1* [out], *入 jap6* [in], *過 gwo3* [past]/[over], *起 hei2* [up], *到 dou3* [arrive at], *番 faan1* [back], with *嚟 lei4* [come] or *去 heoi3* [go], as in *上嚟 soeng5 lei4* 'up come' [come up] and *上去 soeng5 heoi3* 'up go' [go up] (Cheung, 2007, pp. 119–122). Tri-syllabic ones involve a combination of *番 faan1* [back] with the disyllabic ones, as in *番上嚟 faan1 soeng5 lei4* 'back up come' [(come) back up] and *番上去 faan1 soeng5 heoi3* 'back up go' [(go) back up] (Cheung, 2007, pp. 122–123).

Examples

Simple directional particles

拎嚟呢度
ling1 <u>lei4</u> nei1dou6
take come here
(take (it) here)

你幾時飛番香港呀？
nei5 gei2si4 fei1 <u>faan1</u> hoeng1gong2 aa3?
you when fly back Hong Kong SFP
(When will you fly back to Hong Kong?)

Compound directional particles

快啲行上去啦。
faai3 di1 haang4 <u>soeng5 heoi3</u> laa1
fast a-bit walk up go SFP
(Walk up more quickly.)

你跑番過嚟先啦 ！
nei5 paau2 <u>faan1 gwo3 lei4</u> sin1 laa1
you run back over come first SFP
(You run back here first!)

你攞件衫出嚟！
nei5 lo2 gin6 saam1<u>ceot1 lei4</u>
you take CL shirt out come
(You take out the clothes!)

4.3 Potential particles (Pot Prt) 能性助詞

<u>Definition:</u> Potential particles include *得 dak1* [can] and its negative counterpart *唔 m4* [not]. Potential particles typically follow a verb to express the (im)possibility or (in)ability of the situation depicted by the verb phrase being achieved.

Examples

我食得晒啲飯。
ngo5 sik6 <u>dak1</u> saai3 di1 faan6
I eat can all CL rice
(I can finish all the rice.)

我食唔晒啲飯。
ngo5 sik6 <u>m4</u> saai3 di1 faan6
I eat not all CL rice
(I can't finish all the rice.)

4.4 Other verbal particles (Oth VPrt) 其他動詞助詞

<u>**Definition:**</u> We group *親 can1*, *埋 maai4* and *晒 saai3* as other verbal particles. *親 can1* has the adversative meaning when it is used with a transitive verb. *埋 maai4* [also] or [along] denotes the expansion of a domain to bring about the completion of an ongoing action. *晒 saai3* may quantify over the subject of an intransitive verb or the object of a transitive verb to mean [all] or [completely] (Matthews & Yip, 1994, 2011).

Examples

小心，唔好整親隻手呀。
siu2sam1, m4hou2 zing2 <u>can1</u> zek3 sau3 aa3
careful, do-not make PRT CL hand SFP
(Be careful; don't hurt your hand.)

你食埋啲餅先啦！
nei5 sik6 <u>maai4</u> di1 beng2 sin1 laa1
you eat also CL biscuit first SFP
(First, you eat these biscuits too!)

啲人走晒喇。
di1 jan4 zau2 saai3 laa3
CL person leave all SFP
(All the people left.)

佢拎晒啲書番屋企喇。
keoi5 ling1 <u>saai3</u> di1 syu1 faan1 uk1kei2 laa3
s/he take all CL book back home SFP
(S/he took all the books back home.)

5. Complements (Comp) 補語

<u>**Definition:**</u> Complements are phrases that follow the verb phrase to provide additional information about the event depicted by the verb phrase.

5.1 Descriptive complements (Des Comp) 描述補語

<u>**Definition:**</u> Descriptive complements delineate the result or manner of the action or state depicted by a verb or an adjective. The adverbial marker*得 dak1* always

appears between the verb or adjective and the descriptive complement (Cheung, 2007; Matthews & Yip, 1994, 2011).

Examples

佢解釋得好清楚。
keoi5 gaai2sik1 dak1 hou2 cing1co2
s/he explain ADV very clear
(S/he explained very clearly.)

佢真係肥得交關。
keoi5 zan1hai6 fei4 dak1 gaau1gwaan1
s/he really fat ADV extremely
(S/he is so incredibly fat.)

5.2 Complements of extent (Ext Comp) 程度補語

Definition: These complements express the extent of the action or state depicted by a verb or an adjective. *到 dou3* [to the extent] or [until] always appears between the verb or adjective and the complement (Cheung, 2007; Matthews & Yip, 1994, 2011).

Examples

笑到碌地
siu3 dou3 luk1 dei2
laugh to-the-extent trundle floor
(roll on the floor laughing)

佢睇到十點。
keoi5 tai2 dou3 sap6 dim2
s/he see until ten o'clock
(S/he watches (the program) until ten o'clock.)

你今日靚到暈！
nei5 gam1jat6 leng3 dou3 wan4
you today pretty to-the-extent faint
(You look drop-dead gorgeous today!)

5.3 Complements of location (Loc Comp) 處所補語

Definition: These complements indicate the resulting location of the action encoded by the verb.

5.3.1. Localizers (Loc) 方位詞

Definition: Complements of location can appear in the form of a localizer (e.g., 呢度 *nei1dou6* [here], 上面 *soeng6min6* [above], 後面 *hau6min6* [behind]) or a localizer preceded by a noun phrase (e.g., *張枱上面 zoeng1 toi2 soeng6min6* [on top of the table]) (Cheung, 2007; Matthews & Yip, 1994, 2011).

Examples

擺呢度。
baai2 nei1dou6
put here
(Put (it) here.)

擺張枱上面。
baai2 zoeng1 toi2 soeng6min6
put CL table above
(Put (it) on the table.)

5.3.2. Prepositional phrases (PP) 介詞短語

Definition: Complements of location can also appear in the form of a prepositional phrase, with the preposition *喺 hai2* [at] followed by a localizer (e.g., *呢度 nei1dou6* [here] and *嗰度 go2dou6* [there]) or a noun phrase (e.g., *張枱 zoeng1 toi2* [the table]). If the preposition 喺 *hai2* [at] is absent, the sentence is ill formed (Cheung, 2007; Matthews & Yip, 1994, 2011).

Examples

擺架車喺呢度/嗰度。
baai2 gaa3 ce1 hai2 nei1dou6 / go2dou6
put CL car at here / there
(Put the car here/there.)

擺啲書喺張枱度。
baai2 di1 syu1 hai2 zoeng1 toi2 dou6
put CL book at CL table PRT
(Put the books on the table.)

Section C

Sentence Structures (SS)

句子結構

1. Verb-object structure (VO) 動-賓結構

Definition: Verb-object structures consist of a verb that is followed by an object. The verb includes the copula *係 hai6* [be], the existential verb *有 jau5* 'have' [there be] or *冇 mou5* 'not-have' [there not be], In the case of the existential verb, the localizer *呢度 nei1dou6* [here] or *嗰度 go2dou6* [there] in the subject position is dropped. Verb-object structures can be ditransitive constructions with the omission of either the direct or the indirect object and the subject in contexts in which these elements can be recovered.

Examples

攞車車。
lo2 ce1-ce1
take car(-car)
(Take the car.)

係 車車嚟㗎。
hai6 ce1-ce1 lei4 gaa3
be car(-car) SFP SFP
((It) is a car.)

(呢度/嗰度)有 啲蘋果。
(nei1dou6 / go2dou6) jau5 di1 ping4gwo2
(here / there) have(be) CL apple
(There are some apples (here/there).)

俾波波
bei2 bo1bo
give ball
((I) give (Grandma) the ball.)

俾婆婆
bei2 po4po2
give gramma
((I) give Grandma (the ball).

2. Subject-verb-object structure (SVO) 主-動-賓結構

Definition: Subject-verb-object structures contain a subject, a verb (including the copula 係 *hai6* [be]) and an object.

Examples

佢哋 喺度開 禮物呀。
keoi5dei6 hai2dou6 hoi1 lai5mat6 aa3
they ASP open gift SFP
(They are opening the gifts.)

呢個係 我媽媽。
nei1 go3 hai6 ngo5 maa4maa1
this CL be I mother
(This is my mother.)

3. Subject-verb structure (SV) 主語-動詞謂語結構

Definition: Subject-verb structures may consist of 1) a subject and an intransitive verb, 2) a subject and a transitive verb with its object being dropped or 3) a subject and a verb followed by an adjective phrase.

Examples

我瞓覺喇。
ngo5 fan3gaau3 laa3
I sleep SFP
(I am sleeping.)

我洗咗喇。
ngo5 sai2 zo2 laa3
I wash ASP SFP
(I have washed (it.))

我覺得好開心。
ngo5 gok3dak1 hou2 hoi1sam1
I feel very happy
(I feel very happy.)

4. Subject-adjective structure (SA) 主語-形容詞謂語結構

Definition: Subject-adjective structures consist of a subject and an adjective phrase.

Example

我屋企 好細 㗎咋。
ngo5 uk1kei2 hou2 sai3 gaa3 zaa3
I home very small SFP SFP
(My home is very small.)

5. Subject-noun structure (SN) 主語-名詞謂語結構

Definition: Subject-noun structures consist of a subject and a noun phrase.

Example

今日 星期日。
gam1jat6 sing1kei4jat6
today Sunday
(Today is Sunday.)

6. Topic structure (Top) 主題句

Definition: In these structures, the object is moved to a position before the verb to serve as the topic. This process is called object topicalization (Cheung, 2007; Matthew & Yip, 1994, 2011).

Examples

間屋你擺喺上邊呢度。
gaan1 uk1 nei5 baai2 hai2 soeng6bin6 nei1dou6
CL house you put at above here
(You put the house up here.)

啲餅你食埋先啦。
di1 beng2 nei5 sik6 maai4 sin1 laa1
CL biscuit you eat along first SFP
(You eat up the biscuits first.)

7. Existential constructions (EC) 存在句

Definition: In existential constructions, the existential verb *有 jau5* 'have' [there be] and its negative counterpart *冇 mou5* 'not-have' [there not be] are used to introduce a new topic, which may be followed by a verb phrase, a prepositional phrase or other types of phrases (see Matthew & Yip, 1994, 2011).

Examples

好嘢！有雪糕食。
hou2je3! jau5 syut3gou1 sik6
yeah! have ice-cream eat
(Yeah! There is ice cream to eat.)

有隻貓跳咗入嚟。
jau5 zek3 maau1 tiu3 zo2 jap6 lei4
have CL cat jump ASP in come
(A cat jumped in.)

冇人喺公園喎。
mou5 jan4 hai2 gung1jyun2 wo3
not-have person at park SFP
(There is no one at the park.)

8. Comparative constructions (Com C) 比較句

8.1 Comparison of adjectives (Com A) 形容詞的比較

Definition: Several forms of comparison are used, including 啲 *di1* [a bit], *過 gwo3* [than], and *比 bei2* [than]. *比 bei2* [than] is more formal and more commonly used in written text, and it appears before the object and the adjective, in the form of "S *比 bei2* O Adj." The words *太 taai3* [too] and *最 zeoi3* [most] are placed before the adjective to indicate excessive and superlative, respectively (Matthews & Yip, 1994, 2011; see also Cheung, 2007; Tang, 2015).

Examples

哥哥乖啲喎。
go4go1 gwaai1 <u>di1</u> wo3
older-brother well-behaved a-bit SFP
(The older brother is better behaved.)
細佬矮過我。
sai3lou2 ai2 <u>gwo3</u> ngo5
younger-brother short than I
(My younger brother is shorter than me.)

8.2 Comparing quantities (Com Qua) 數量的比較

<u>Definition:</u> When comparing quantities, *多 do1* [much/many] and *少 siu2* [little/few], which also mean [more] and [less/fewer], respectively, are used in comparative constructions with 過 *gwo3* [than] or *比 bei2* [than] (Matthews & Yip, 2011).

Example

我貼紙多過你。
ngo5 tip3zi2 <u>do1 gwo3</u> nei5
I sticker more than you
(I have more stickers than you.)

9. Pivotal constructions (PC) 兼語結構

<u>Definition:</u> Pivotal constructions involve a noun phrase, which simultaneously serves as the object of the first verb and the subject of the second verb (Cheung, 2007). A small set of verbs can go in as the first verb of a pivotal construction. One such verb is the permissive *俾 bei2* [allow].

Examples

我揀佢做班長。
<u>ngo5 gaan2</u> <u>keoi5 zou6</u> baan1zoeng2
I choose s/he do class-representative
(I choose him/her to be the class representative.)

我唔俾 佢睇電視。
<u>ngo5 m4 bei2</u> <u>keoi5 tai2</u> din6si6
I not allow s/he see TV
(I do not let him/her watch TV.)

10. Passive structure (Pass) 被動句

<u>Definition:</u> Similar to Mandarin, Cantonese has a passive structure with the word *俾 bei2* introducing the agent of the action, which is followed by a verb phrase.

Unlike Mandarin *被 bèi* passives, the presence of the agent is obligatory in Cantonese (Matthews & Yip, 2011).

Example

弟弟俾姐姐嘈醒咗。
dai4dai2 bei2 ze4ze1 cou4 seng2 zo2
younger-brother by older-sister make-noise awake ASP
(The younger brother was awakened by the noise the older sister made.)

11. 將 zoeng1 construction (ZC) 「將」字句

Definition: Like the Mandarin *把 bǎ* construction, Cantonese has a counterpart marked by *將 zoeng1*. *將 zoeng1* takes a noun phrase, which is the object of the following verb phrase. However, unlike Mandarin *把 bǎ*, *將 zoeng1* is not used with all transitive verbs (Matthews & Yip, 2011).

Example

將啲蕃茄放落去煮。
zoeng1 di1 faan1ke2 fong3 lok6 heoi3 zyu2
PREP CL tomato put down go cook
(Put the tomatoes into (something) to cook (them).)

12. Sentences with a prepositional phrase (S PP) 包含介詞短語的句子

Definition: A prepositional phrase, which consists of a preposition and a noun phrase, usually appears before the verb, with the exception of the *俾 bei2*-construction (Cheung, 2007). Prepositions are also referred to as coverbs (Matthews & Yip, 1994, 2011).

12.1 *俾 bei2* construction 俾」字句

Definition: When the main verb is a dative verb (e.g., *拎 ling2* [take]) encoding transfer of objects, the construction in which the *俾 bei2* prepositional phrase appears is also called a prepositional dative construction. The preposition *俾 bei2* is often translated as 'for' or 'to' in English (Tang, 2015).

Examples

開電視俾你睇。
hoi1 din6si6 bei2 nei5 tai2
turn-on TV for you see
(Turn on the TV for you to see.)

我寫咗張卡俾佢。
ngo5 se2 zo2 zoeng1 kaat1 bei2 keoi5
I write ASP CL card to s/he
(I have written a card to him/her.)

拎條褲俾我吖唔該。
ling1 tiu4 fu3 <u>bei2</u> ngo5 aa1 m4goi1
bring CL pants to I SFP thank-you
(Please bring the pants to me.)

12.2 *喺 hai2* construction 「喺」字句

<u>Definition:</u> In this construction, the preposition phrase with *喺 hai2* [at] may be followed by a verb phrase or it may appear alone. The preposition *喺 hai2* [at] may appear before the localizer *度 dou6* [here], and together they function as a prepositional phrase *喺度 hai2dou6* 'at here' [here].

Examples

佢喺泳池游水
keoi5 <u>hai2</u> wing6ci4 jau4seoi2
s/he at swimming-pool swim
(S/he swims at the swimming pool.)

佢喺泳池。
keoi5 <u>hai2</u> wing6ci4
s/he at swimming-pool
(S/he is at the swimming pool.)

我<u>喺度</u>呀。
ngo5 <u>hai2dou6</u> aa3
I at-here SFP
(I am here.)

我<u>喺度</u>做功課。★
ngo5 <u>hai2dou6</u> zou6 gung1fo3
I at-here/ASP do homework
(I do my homework here.)
(I am doing my homework.)

★ The use of *喺度 hai2dou6* is ambiguous here. It can mean [at here], or it can be an imperfective aspect marker, depending on the context.

12.3 *對 deoi3* construction「對」字句

<u>Definition:</u> The preposition *對 deoi3* is often translated as 'to' or 'towards' in English.

Example

隻狗對住個賊吠。
zek3 gau2 <u>deoi3</u> zyu6 go3 caak2 fai6
CL dog towards ASP CL thief bark
(The dog barks at the thief.)

12.4 *同 tung4* construction 「同」字句

Definition: The preposition *同 tung4* is often translated as 'with' or 'together with' in English. Note that *同 tung4* can function as a verb in other contexts meaning *幫 bong1* [help].

Example

我同佢哋玩。
ngo5 tung4 keoi5dei6 waan2
I with they play
(I play with them.)

12.5 *到 dou3* construction 「到」字句

Definition: *到 dou3* means [to be followed by] when followed by a pronoun or a noun and [until] or [by] when followed by a temporal expression.

Examples

到你玩喇！
dou3 nei5 waan2 laa3
to-be-followed-by you play SFP
(It's your turn to play!)

到而家你都仲未起身呀？
dou3 ji4gaa1 nei5 dou1 zung6 mei6 hei2san1 aa4
by now you also still not-yet get-up SFP
(You still haven't got up yet?)

13. Clausal complements (CC) 賓語從句

Definition: Clausal complements are clauses that appear after verbs of perception (e.g., *見 gin3* [see], *聽 teng1* [hear]) or mental state terms (e.g., *諗 lam2* [think], *估 gu2* [guess]). The last example illustrates an infinitival clause in which an overt subject is absent.

Examples

我見到有人喺門口行過。
ngo5 gin3 dou2 jau5 jan4 hai2 mun4hau2 haang4 gwo3
I see PRT have person at doorway walk past
(I saw someone/some people walk past the door.)

我諗佢多數都係唔嚟㗎喇。
ngo5 lam2 keoi5 do1sou3 dou1 hai6 m4 lei4 gaa3 laa3
I think s/he probably also be not come SFP SFP
(I think s/he probably is not coming.)

我真係唔明白佢點解咁樣做。
ngo5 zan1hai6 m4 ming4baak6 keoi5 dim2gaai2 gam2joeng2 zou6
I really not understand s/he why like-this do
(I really don't understand why s/he did this.)

我覺得佢好開心喎。
ngo5 gok3dak1 keoi5 hou2 hoi1sam1 wo3
I feel s/he very happy SFP
(I feel s/he is very happy.)

我哋而家開始食早餐喇！
ngo5dei2 ji4gaa1 hoi1ci2 sik6 zou2caan1 laa3
we now begin eat breakfast SFP
(We begin to eat breakfast now!)

14. Serial verb constructions (SVC) 連動結構

Definition: A serial verb construction (SVC) contains two or more verbs sharing the same subject, with no intervening conjunctions, fillers (e.g., *哩 le1*) or pause between the verbs. It depicts a single event that is composed of sub-events. Reversal of the order of the verb phrases inside an SVC will lead to a change of meaning or ill formedness. The SVC types illustrated next are classified in terms of the semantic notions that the constituent verbs convey (Fung, 2011; Matthews, 2006). They are not intended to be exhaustive.

14.1 Serial verb constructions: Simple (SVC-1) 簡單連動結構

I. Benefactive 施惠

Definition: Benefactive SVCs convey the meaning of helping or conferring benefits to someone. The verb *幫 bong1* [help] is typically used to introduce the beneficiary, but *同 tung4* [help] can also be used when it functions as a verb.

Examples

我幫你 洗咗啲碗啦。
ngo5 bong1 nei5 sai2 zo2 di1 wun2 laa1
I help you wash ASP CL bowl SFP
(Let me help you wash the dishes.)

我同你 整番好架車喇。
ngo5 tung4 nei5 zing2 faan1 hou2 gaa3 ce1 laa3
I help you make back good CL car SFP
(I helped you repair the car.)

II. Comitative 伴隨

Definition: Comitative SVCs involve the notion of companionship. *陪 pui4* [accompany] is typically used to introduce the individual being accompanied by the agent. The word *帶 daai3* [bring] can also be used for this type of serial verb construction.

Example

媽咪琴日陪/帶我去公園。
maa1mi4 kam4jat6 pui4 / daai3 ngo5 heoi3 gung1jyun2
mommy yesterday accompany / bring I go park
(Mommy accompanied/brought me to the park yesterday.)

III. Instrumental 工具性

Definition: Instrumental SVCs encode actions that change an object from one state to another through the use of an instrument (Luke & Bodomo, 2001). *攞 lo2* [take], *用 jung6* [use], and *搵 wan2* [find] are typically used to introduce the instrument used to carry out the action encoded by the second verb. The instrument that goes between the first verb and the second verb is sometimes omitted or moved to the subject position when the verb is *嚟 lei4* [come] (e.g., *愛嚟 oi3lei4* 'love-come,' *攞嚟 lo2lei4* 'take-come' and *用嚟 jung6lei4* 'use-come'), which is then followed by another verb that specifies the action performed through the use of the instrument (Fung, 2011).

Examples

佢用呢條鎖匙 開門。
keoi5 jung6 nei1 tiu4 so2si4 hoi1 mun4
s/he use this CL key open door
(S/he uses this key to open the door.)

愛嚟 洗面
oi3lei4 sai2 min6
love-come wash face
(used for washing (your) face)

呢個用嚟 切嘢。
nei1 go3 jung6lei4 cit3 je5
this CL use-come cut thing
(This is used for cutting.)

IV. Directional 方位

Definition: Directional SVCs convey the meaning of "deixis, directionality or movement towards/from a certain direction" (Luke & Bodomo, 2001, p. 176). Unlike Fung (2011), directional SVCs here do not require the first verb to be a directional verb (e.g., *出 ceot1* [out], *入 jap6* [in], *上 seong5* [up], *落 lok6* [down], *過 gwo3* [past], *返 faan1* [return]) or the second verb to be a deictic verb *去 heoi3* [go] or *嚟 lei4* [come]. Instead, the first verb must be followed by a noun phrase, and the actions denoted by the first and the second verb must be carried out by the same agent.[1]

Example

你攞件衫 返屋企。
nei5 lo2 gin6 saam1 faan1 uk1kei2
you take CL shirt return home
(You take the shirt and return home.)

V. Purpose 目的

Definition: In Purpose SVCs, the first verb denotes an action, and the subsequent verbs express the purpose of that action. The first verb can be a deictic verb (e.g., 去 *heoi3* [go], 嚟 *lei4* [come]), and in such cases, the noun phrase that goes between the first and the second verb can be omitted. The first verb can also be a verb other than a deictic verb (Fung, 2011).

Examples

我去(書店) 買書。
ngo5 heoi3 (syu1dim3) maai5 syu1
I go (bookstore) buy book
(I go (to the bookstore) to buy books.)

買本書 (嚟) 睇吓。
maai5 bun2 syu1 (lei4) tai2 haa5
buy CL book (come) see ASP
((Let me) buy a book to read.)

VI. Sequential 順序

Definition: Sequential SVCs encode actions that are performed consecutively in a sequence. The order of the verbs corresponds to the order of the actions encoded by the verbs. The perfective aspect marker is often used to mark the completion of the first action (Fung, 2011).

Examples

佢除咗對鞋 入屋。
keoi5 ceoi4 zo2 deoi3 haai4 jap6 uk1
s/he remove ASP pair shoe enter house
(S/he removed his/her shoes and then entered the house.)

佢入屋除咗對鞋。
keoi5 jap6 uk1 ceoi4 zo2 deoi3 haai4
s/he enter house remove ASP pair shoe
(S/he entered the house and then removed his/her shoes.)

VII. Alternating 往復

Definition: Alternating SVCs encode actions that occur to and from in alternation (Fung, 2011).

Example

佢喺度行嚟 行去。
keoi5 hai2dou6 haang4-lei4-haang4-heoi3
s/he ASP walk-come-walk-go
(S/he is walking around.)

VIII. Circumstance 情境

Definition: Circumstance SVCs require the first verb to describe a circumstance under which the action denoted by the second verb takes place (Fung, 2011).

Example

搭地鐵 睇書
daap3 dei6tit3 tai2 syu1
ride subway see book
(read while taking the subway)

IX. Posture 姿態

Definition: Posture SVCs require the first verb to describe the posture of the action depicted by the second verb. The first verb is often followed by the aspect marker 住 *zyu6* (Fung, 2011).

Example

佢瞓住 睇書。
keoi5 fan3 zyu6 tai2 syu1
s/he lie-down ASP see book
(S/he is reading a book while lying down.)

14.2 Serial verb constructions: complex (SVC-2) 複雜連動結構

Definition: SVCs can become more complex when they involve more than one semantic type of SVC.

Examples

Comitative and purpose

爸爸陪細佬 去7–11 買雪糕。
ba4ba1 pui4 sai3lou2 heoi3 7–11 maai5 syut3gou1
father accompany younger-brother go 7–11 buy ice-cream
(Dad accompanies the younger brother to go to 7–11 to buy ice cream.)

Instrumental and purpose

佢用條梯 爬上去 攞個波。
keoi5 jung6 tiu4 tai1 paa4 soeng5 heoi3 lo2 go3 bo1
S/he use CL ladder climb up go get CL ball
(S/he uses a ladder to climb up (there) to get the ball.)

15. Complex sentences without overt conjunctions (CS-Conj) 無連詞複句

Definition: Complex sentences are sentences that contain two or more clauses. These clauses can be linked by one conjunction or two conjunctions working in pair. (See Section E2 for an illustration of the conjunctions.) Clauses can also be put together to express different kinds of semantic relations without overt conjunctions. In the following example, there is a causal relation between the two clauses that is not marked by an explicit conjunction.

Example

出邊好大雨, 你唔可以踩單車㗎。
ceot1bin6 hou2 daai6 jyu5, nei5 m4 ho2ji5 caai2 daan1ce1 gaa3
outside very big rain, you not can ride bike SPF
(Because it is raining heavily outside, you cannot ride your bike.)

Section D

Questions

疑問句

1. Yes/no questions (YN) 是非問句

Definition: There are eight types of yes/no questions. They are particle questions, A-not-A questions, copula questions, *未 mei6* questions, existential questions, tag questions, intonation questions and echo questions (Matthews & Yip, 1994, 2011).

1.1 Particle questions (Prt Q) 助詞問句

Definition: Particle questions are the simplest question type formed by adding one or sometimes two particles to a declarative sentence (Matthews & Yip, 1994, 2011).

Example

你唔知嘅咩？
nei5 m4 zi1 ge3 me1
you not know SFP SFP
(Don't you know?)

1.2 A-not-A questions (A Q) 正反問句

<u>Definition:</u> This form of question involves repetition of the first syllable of a verb or adjective, with the negative morpheme *唔 m4* [not] appearing between them (Matthews & Yip, 1994, 2011; Law, 2001).

Example

你<u>鍾唔鍾意</u>食糖呀？
nei5 <u>zung1-m4-zung1ji3</u> sik6 tong2 aa3
you like-not-like-to eat candy SFP
(Do you like eating candies?)

1.3 Copula questions (Cop Q) 「係咪」問句

<u>Definition:</u> Copula questions are marked by the copular verb *係 hai6* [be] in the A-not-A form *係唔係 hai6m4hai6* 'be-not-be,' which precedes the main verb. *係咪 hai6mai6* is a contracted form of *係唔係 hai6m4hai6* (Matthews & Yip, 1994, 2011).

Example

你<u>係咪</u>要呀？
nei5 <u>hai6mai6</u> jiu3 aa3
you be-not-be want SFP
(Do you want it?)

1.4 *未 mei6* questions (*未 mei6* Q) 「未」問句

<u>Definition:</u> This form of question involves the addition of the negative morpheme *未 mei6* [not-yet] to a declarative sentence to form a question asking whether an event has taken place or not (Matthews & Yip, 1994, 2011).

Example

你食咗飯<u>未</u>呀？
nei5 sik6 zo2 faan6 <u>mei6</u> aa3
you eat ASP rice not-yet SFP
(Have you had your meal yet?)

1.5 Existential questions (Exi Q) 存在問句

<u>Definition:</u> Existential questions use the words *有冇 jau5mou5* 'have-not-have (there-be-not-be)' to ask whether something exists or not (Matthews & Yip, 1994, 2011).

Example

呢度<u>有冇</u>車車呀？
nei1dou6 <u>jau5mou5</u> ce1-ce1 aa3
here have-not-have *car(-car)* SFP
(Is there a car here?)

1.6 Tag questions (Tag Q) 附加問句

Definition: Tag questions are used to turn statements into questions. The tag is attached at the end of a statement. Some common tags are *係唔係 hai6-m4-hai6* 'be-not-be,' *好唔好 hou2-m4-hou2* 'good-not-good' and *得唔得 dak1-m4-dak1* 'can-not-can' (Matthews & Yip, 1994, 2011).

Example

你唔去喇，係唔係呀？
nei5 m4 heoi3 laa3, hai6-m4-hai6 aa3
you not go SFP, be-not-be SFP
(You are not going, are you?)

1.7 Intonation questions (Int Q) 語調問句

Definition: Intonation questions are questions marked by a rising intonation alone (Matthews & Yip, 1994, 2011).

Example

你真係唔食？
nei5 zan1hai6 m4 sik6
you really not eat
(You're really not eating (this)?)

1.8 Echo questions (Ech Q) 反問問句

Definition: Echo questions are questions marked by rising intonation alone or the sentence final particle *話 waa6* [huh] (Matthews & Yip, 1994, 2011). These questions are used when the speaker repeats a statement out of surprise or disbelief.

Examples

你唔嚟？
nei5 m4 lei4
you not come
(You are not coming?)

你食咗咩話？
nei5 sik6 zo2 me1 waa2
you eat ASP what huh
(What did you say you have eaten, huh?)

2. *Wh*-questions (WhQ) 特指問句

Definition: As a *wh*-in-situ language, Cantonese allows its *wh* words to stay in situ. For instance, the *wh* word *邊個 bin1go3* [who] may serve as a subject or an object, which differs from English, in which the *wh* words always appear at the beginning of the sentence (Matthews & Yip, 1994, 2011). The *wh* words in Section 2.1 are observed in children before 30 months (Frank et al., 2017; Tardif et al., 2008), and those in 2.2 appear after 30 months.

Examples

Subject question

邊個搵我呀？
bin1go3 wan2 ngo5 aa3
who find I SFP
(Who is looking for me?)

Object question

你搵邊個呀？
nei5 wan2 bin1go3 aa3
you find who SFP
(Who are you looking for?)

2.1 Wh words (Wh-1) 疑問代詞

I. "What" questions – 乜嘢 mat1je5/咩 me1 「乜嘢/咩」疑問句

Example

呢個咩嚟㗎？
nei1 go3 me1 lei4 gaa3
this CL what SFP SFP
(What is this?)

II. "Who" question – 邊個 bin1go3 「邊個」疑問句

Example

幅畫邊個畫㗎？
fuk1 waa2 bin1go3 waak6 gaa3
CL picture who draw SFP
(Who drew this picture?)

III. "Where" questions – 邊度 bin1dou6/邊庶 bin1syu3/邊 bin1 「邊度/邊庶/邊」疑問句

Example

擺喺邊度呢？
baai2 hai2 bin1dou6 le1
put at where SFP
(Where do (I) put (this)?)

IV. "Why" and reason questions – 做乜 zou6mat1/做咩 zou6me1/做乜嘢 zou6mat1je5/點解 dim2gaai2 「做乜/做咩/做乜嘢/點解」疑問句

Example

做乜有一個橙嘅？
zou6mat1 jau5 jat1 go3 caang2 ge2
why have one CL orange SFP
(Why is there one orange?)

Note: The use of the *wh* word *點解 dim2gaai2* [why] for "why" questions comes later than 30 months.

2.2 Wh words (Wh-2) 疑問代詞

I. "Which" questions – 邊 *bin1* + CL 「邊 + 名量詞」疑問句

Example

你想要邊部車呀？
nei5 soeng2jiu3 bin1 bou6 ce1 aa3
you want which CL car SFP
(Which car do you want?)

II. "How many/much" questions – 幾多 gei2do1 「幾多」疑問句

Example

有幾多架車呀？
jau5 gei2do1 gaa3 ce1 aa3
have how-many CL car SFP
(How many cars are there?)

III. "When" and time questions – 幾時 gei2si4 「幾時」疑問句

Example

幾時返課室呀？
gei2si4 faan1 fo3sat1 aa3
when return classroom SFP
(When do (we) return to the classroom?)

IV. "How" questions – 點樣 dim2joeng2/點 dim2 「點樣/點」疑問句

Example

點樣摺飛機㗎？
dim2joeng2 zip3 fei1gei1 gaa3
how fold airplane SFP
(How do (I) fold an airplane?)

Section E

Sentence adverbs, conjunctions and sentence final particles

修飾句子的副詞、連詞、句末助詞

1. Sentence adverbs (S Adv) 修飾句子的副詞

Definition: Sentence adverbs serve to modify the whole sentence (Matthews & Yip, 1994, 2011). They include scope adverbs, temporal adverbs, frequency adverbs and modal adverbs (Matthews & Yip, 1994, 2011). Typically, they may appear at the beginning of the sentence or between the subject and the verb phrase or adjective phrase. Occasionally, some of them may appear at the end of the sentence, by way of an afterthought.

1.1 Scope adverbs (Sco Adv) 範圍副詞

Definition: Scope adverbs are used to specify the scope and quantity in which the event depicted by the sentence takes effect. Examples are 淨係 *zing6hai6* [only], *差啲 caa1di1* [almost], 都 *dou1* [also]/[too], *冚唪唥 ham6baang6laang6* [all] and *爭少少 zaang1syu2syu2* [almost] (Cheung, 2007; Wong, 2002).

Examples

淨係黃老師教我哋英文㗎咋。
zing6hai6 wong4 lou5si1 gaau3 ngo5dei6 jing1man2 gaa3 zaa3
only Wong teacher teach we English SFP SFP
(Only Miss Wong teaches us English.)

黃老師淨係教我哋英文㗎咋。
wong4 lou5si1 zing6hai6 gaau3 ngo5dei6 jing1man2 gaa3 zaa3
Wong teacher only teach we English SFP SFP
(Miss Wong only teaches us English.)

我差啲認唔到佢。
ngo5 caa1di1 jing6 m4 dou2 keoi5
I almost recognize not PRT s/he
(I almost can't recognize him/her.)

A: *我鍾意朱古力。*
ngo5 zung1ji3 zyu1gu1lik1
I like chocolate
(I like chocolate.)

B: *我都係呀。*
ngo5 dou1 hai6 aa3
I also be SFP
(I like it too.)

1.2 Temporal adverbs (Tem Adv) 時間副詞

<u>Definition:</u> Temporal adverbs indicate the time or duration during which the event described by the sentence takes place. Examples include *依家 ji1gaa1/而家 ji4gaa1* [now], *頭先 tau4sin1/啱啱 ngaam1ngaam1* [just now], *下次 haa6ci3* [next time], *以前 ji5cin4/之前 zi1cin4* [before], *一陣間 jat1zan6gaan1* [in a moment], *嗰陣時 go2zan6si4* [that time]/[formerly], *仲 zung6* [still], *先 sin1/先至 sin1zi3* [only then], *首先 sau2sin1* [first of all], *先 sin1* [first], *已經 ji5ging1* [already], *即刻 zik1hak1* [immediately] and *就 zau6/就嚟 zau6lei4/就快 zau6faai3* [soon]/[almost] (Cheung, 2007; Matthews & Yip, 1994, 2011; Wong, 2002).

Examples

<u>嗰陣時</u>我<u>仲</u>未學畫畫。
<u>go2zan6si4</u> ngo5 <u>zung6</u> mei6 hok6 waak6 waa2
that-time I still not-yet learn draw picture
(At that time, I still hadn't learned to paint.)

我<u>仲</u>要多一碗飯呀，唔該。`12
ngo5 <u>zung6</u> jiu3 do1 jat1 wun2 faan6 aa3, m4goi1
I still want more one bowl rice SFP, thank-you
(I still want one more bowl of rice, please.)

咁樣整<u>先至</u>可以攞佢入嚟。
gam2joeng2 zing2 <u>sin1zi3</u> ho2ji5 lo2 keoi5 jap6 lei4
like-this make only-then can bring it enter come
((You) can bring it in only if (you) do this.)

我哋<u>先</u>影咗佢<u>再</u>算。
ngo5dei6 <u>sin1</u> jing2 zo2 keoi5 <u>zoi3</u> syun3
we first take-a-photo ASP s/he after-that count(think)
(Let's take a photo of him/her first and then consider the next step.)

我<u>就</u>到喇。
ngo5 <u>zau6</u> dou3 laa3
I soon arrive SFP
(I'm arriving soon.)

1.3 Frequency adverbs (Fre Adv) 頻率副詞

<u>Definition:</u> Frequency adverbs indicate the frequency or repetitiveness of the event described by the sentence. Examples include *又 jau6/又試 jau6si3* [again], *再 zoi3* [once again], *通常 tung1soeng4* [usually], *好少 hou2siu2/好少可 hou2siu2ho2* [rarely], *成日 seng4jat6* 'all-day' [often], *每次 mui5ci3* [every time] and *日日 jat6jat6* [every day] (Matthews & Yip, 2011; Wong, 2002).

Examples

佢又遲到喇今日。
keoi5 jau6 ci4dou3 laa3 kam1jat6
s/he again late-arrive SFP today
(S/he is late again today.)

爸爸好少咁早返嚟㗎。
baa4baa1 hou2siu2 gam3 zou2 faan1 lei4 gaa3
daddy rarely this early return come SFP
(Daddy rarely comes back this early.)

1.4 Modal adverbs (Mod Adv) 語氣副詞

Definition: Modal adverbs describe the possibility, likelihood, certainty of the event (e.g., *多數 do1sou3* [probably], *可能 ho2nang4* [maybe], *梗係 gang-2hai6* [bound to]/[surely], *絕對 zyut6deoi3* [absolutely] and *一定 jat1ding6/肯定 hang2ding6* [surely]) (Cheung, 2007; Matthews & Yip, 1994, 2011; Wong, 2002). They also indicate the speaker's attitude towards the event (e.g., *居然 geoi1jin4/竟然 ging2jin4* (expressing unexpectedness or surprise)) (Cheung, 2007; Wong, 2002) or point of view (e.g., *大體上 daai6tai2soeng6/整體上 zing2tai2soeng6* [on the whole]/[overall], *大致上 daai6zi3soeng6* [approximately]/[roughly], *聽講(話) tenglgong2(waa6)* [by hearsay]/[allegedly] and *好似(係) hou2ci5(hai6)* [seemingly]/[vaguely]) (Matthews & Yip, 1994, 2011; Wong, 2002).

Example

佢多數都係唔嚟㗎喇。
keoi5 do1sou3 dou1 hai6 m4 lei4 gaa3 laa3
s/he probably also be not come SFP SFP
(S/he is probably not going to come.)

2. Conjunctions (Conj) 連詞

Definition: Conjunctions are used to join words, phrases or clauses together. Here, we only include conjunctions for phrases and clauses. There are different types of conjunctions indicating different semantic relations: coordinating, causal, concessive, conditional, temporal and purposive. Some conjunctions appear in pairs.

2.1 Coordinating conjunctions (Coor Conj) 並列連詞

(e.g., 又 . . . 又 . . . *jau6 . . . jau6* . . . 'also . . . also . . .' [. . . and . . .], 一係 . . . 一係 . . . *jat1hai6 . . . jat1hai6* . . . 'either . . . either . . .' [either . . . or . . .], . . . 或者 . . . *waak6ze2* . . . [. . . or . . .]) (Matthews & Yip, 1994, 2011).

Examples

你又想玩車，又想玩波，唔得㗎噃。
nei5 jau6 soeng2 waan2 ce1, jau6 soeng2 waan2 bo1, m4 dak1 gaa3 bo3
you also want-to play car, also want-to play ball, not can SFP SFP
(You want to play with the car, and (you) also want to play with the ball. It doesn't work like that.)

你一係煮飯一係掃地。
nei5 jat1hai6 zyu2faan6 jat1hai6 sou3 dei6
you either cook-rice either sweep floor
(You either cook or sweep the floor.)

2.2 Causal conjunctions (Caus Conj) 因果連詞

(e.g., . . . 因爲 . . . *jan1wai6* . . . [. . . because . . .], . . . 所以 . . . *so2ji5* . . . [. . . so/therefore . . .]) (Matthews & Yip, 1994, 2011).

Example

因爲冇鬧鐘囉。
jan1wai6 mou5 naau6zung1 lo1
because not-have alarm-clock SFP
(Because (I) have no alarm clock.)

2.3 Concession conjunctions (Conc Conj) 轉折連詞

(e.g., 雖然 . . . 但係 . . . *seoi1jin4* . . . *daan6hai6* . . . 'although . . . but . . .' [although . . .], . . . 但係 . . . *daan6hai6* . . . [. . . but . . .], 雖然 . . . 都 . . . *seoi1jin4* . . . *dou1* . . . 'although . . . still/also . . .' [although . . . still . . .], 無論 . . . 都 . . . *mou4leon4* . . . *dou1* . . . [no matter . . . still/also . . .]) (Matthews & Yip, 1994, 2011).

Examples

但係我唔想返屋企。
daan6hai6 ngo5 m4 soeng2 faan1 uk1kei2
but I not want-to return home
(But I don't want to go back home.)

佢雖然好高，
keoi5 seoi1jin4 hou2 gou1,
s/he although very tall,

但係 都攞唔到喺櫃上邊個樽。
daan6hai6 dou1 lo2 m4 dou2 hai2 gwai6 soeng6bin6 go3 zeon1
but still take not PRT at cupboard above CL bottle
(Although s/he is very tall, (s/he) still cannot reach the bottle on top of the cupboard.)

2.4 Conditional conjunctions (Cond Conj) 條件連詞

(e.g., 如果 . . . 就 . . . *jyu4gwo2 . . . zau6 . . .* [if . . . then . . .], 就算 . . . 都 . . . *zau6syun3 . . . dou1 . . .* [even if . . . still . . .]) (Matthews & Yip, 1994, 2011).

Example

如果病咗，就要去睇醫生。
jyu4gwo2 beng6 zo2, zau6 jiu3 heoi3 tai2 ji1sang1
if sick ASP, then need-to go see doctor
(If (one) is sick, then (one) has to go see a doctor.)

2.5 Temporal conjunctions (Temp Conj) 時間連詞

(e.g., . . . 嗰陣時 . . . *go2zan6si4*/. . . 嗰陣 . . . *go2zan6* '. . . that-time' [the time when . . .], . . . 嘅時候 . . . *ge3si4hau6* '. . . PRT-time (the-time-of . . .)' [the time when . . .], . . . 之前 . . . *zi1cin4* [before . . .], . . . 之後 . . . *zi1hau6* [after . . .], 一路 . . . 一路 . . . *jat1lou6 . . . jat1lou6 . . .* 'one time . . . one time . . .' [. . . while . . .]) (Matthews & Yip, 1994, 2011).

Examples

妹妹一路睇電視一路做功課。
mui4mui2 jat1lou6 tai2 din6si6 jat1lou6 zou6 gung1fo3
younger-sister one-time watch TV one-time do homework
(The younger sister is watching television while doing her homework.)

老師講嘢嘅時候，我哋要安靜。
lou5si1 gong2 je5 ge3si4hau6, ngo5dei6 jiu3 on1zing6
teacher speak thing PRT-time, we need-to quiet
(When the teacher speaks, we need to be quiet.)

我細個嗰陣時，成日去海洋公園玩㗎。
ngo5 sai3 go3 go2zan6si4, seng4jat6 heoi3 hoi2joeng4gung1jyun2 waan2 gaa2
I small CL that-time, often go Ocean-Park play SFP
(When I was small, I often went to Ocean Park to play.)

你做完功課先再去玩。
nei5 zou6 jyun4 gong1fo3 sin1 joi3 heoi3 waan2
you do finish homework first after-that go play
(You finish doing your homework first, and then (you) go play.)

畫完畫之後去飲茶。
waak6 jyun4 waa2 zi1hau6 heoi3 jam2caa4
draw finish picture after go drink-tea (yum-cha)
((Let's) go to yum-cha after (we) finish painting.)

2.6 Purpose conjunctions (Purp Conj) 目的連詞

(e.g., 爲咗 . . . *wai6zo2 . . .* 'for' [in order to]/[for the purpose that]) (Matthews & Yip, 1994, 2011)

Example

爲咗要佢開心我乜嘢都肯做。
wai6zo2 jiu3 keoi5 hoi1sam1 ngo5 mat1je5 dou1 hang2 zou6
for want s/he happy I what(ever) also willing-to do
(I am willing to do anything to make him/her happy.)

3. Sentence final particles (SFP) 句末助詞

Definition: Sentence final particles (also referred to as utterance particles (Luke, 1990)) serve various semantic and communicative functions, such as indicating the speech-act types (e.g., assertions, questions, requests) and evidentiality (i.e., the source of knowledge) of the sentence, as well as expressing the speaker's attitudes, moods and emotions towards the situation (Matthews & Yip, 1994, 2011; Tang, 2015; see also Fung, 2000; Kwok, 1984; Law, 1990; Luke, 1990). They can appear in isolation or in combination (e.g., *㗎喇噃 gaa3laa3bo3*) at the end of a sentence. The same particle can carry different tones (e.g., *呀 aa1, aa3* (could be written as *吖 for aa1*)) and, hence, convey different functions and meanings.

Examples

我唔會去呀。
ngo5 m4 wui5 heoi3 aa3
I not will go SFP
(I will not go).

咁熱嘅。
gam3 jit6 ge2
so hot SFP
(It's so hot!)

係兔仔嚟㗎。
hai6 tou3zai2 lei4 gaa3
be rabbit SFP SFP
(It's a rabbit!)

睇吓你點整先。
tai2 haa5 nei5 dim2 zing2 sin1
see ASP you how make SFP
((Let's) see how you do it.)

仲可以玩玩具添。
zung6 ho2ji5 waan2 wun6geoi6 tim1
also may play toy SFP
((We) may play with toys too.)

Note

1 In the following example, 出嚟 *ceot1 lei4* 'out come' is analyzed as a compound directional particle. The sentence is not considered an SVC because the action 攞 *lo2* [take] is carried out by you, and the movement 出嚟 *ceot1 lei4* 'out come' involves not you but the clothes.

3

THE DEVELOPMENT OF GRAMMAR IN CANTONESE-SPEAKING PRESCHOOL CHILDREN

Chapter 1 gives a descriptive overview of the adult end-state of grammatical development in Cantonese. From the overview, it is clear that there is a lot about Cantonese grammar for a young child to learn. Research with English-speaking children has shown that children learn the various aspects of the language(s) they are exposed to gradually over time (e.g., Brown, 1973; Fletcher, 1985; Wells, 1986). Questions that naturally arise for speech-language therapists, educators and child language researchers working with Cantonese-speaking children may include the following: Are there valid measures that capture grammatical development across age? What are the age and order of development of different grammatical forms and structures? What kind of grammatical forms and structures do we observe in children as they produce longer sentences? In this chapter, we will address these questions by analyzing the cross-sectional HKU-70X conversational samples and longitudinal conversation samples from one of the eight children in the CANCORP, using the *Grammatical Analysis of Cantonese* (GACS) framework described in Chapter 2. We will relate our findings from the quantitative and qualitative analyses to the existing literature.

3.1 The Hong Kong language context

The development of grammar is shaped by the language context of the home and the community at large. As we refer to language samples collected from Cantonese-speaking children in Hong Kong, a brief discussion on the city's language context is appropriate here. According to the 2016 population bi-census (Census and Statistics Department, 2017), Cantonese is spoken by 88.9% of the population aged five and above at home, compared to 90.8% in 2006 (Census and Statistics Department, 2007). Despite the slight drop, Cantonese continues to be the community language in which people in the city conduct their daily business and

DOI: 10.4324/9780367824013-3

socialize. During the same ten-year period, there was an increase in the percentage of the population aged five and above who could speak Mandarin from 40.2% to 48.6% (Census and Statistics Department, 2017). A similar increase was reported in speakers who could use English as the usual spoken language or an additional language, from 44.7% to 53.2% (Census and Statistics Department, 2017). These trends were not unexpected. Hong Kong was a British colony until the handover of its sovereignty back to China in 1997. Since 1997, English has remained an official language, and the Hong Kong Special Administration Government promotes "biliterate and trilingual" competence in its citizens through various policy initiatives. Children are taught English and/or Mandarin to various extents as early as three years of age through kindergarten, which virtually all children between three and five years old (Hong Kong Government, 2021) attend either half-day or full day. In addition, in Hong Kong, 13.4% households employed a domestic helper (Census and Statistics Department, 2021), and a majority of these helpers are from either the Philippines or Indonesia. While domestic helpers who have been in Hong Kong for a long time might speak some Cantonese, many of them use English. Therefore, some children have additional exposure to English at home as well, albeit from a non-native speaker.

The dynamic language context in Hong Kong at home and at school can have an impact on children's development of the various aspects of Cantonese, including vocabulary, grammar and pragmatics. Here is an example on grammar. One of the children in the CANCORP, LTF, exclusively used the 喺 *hai2* [at] prepositional phrase after the verb (i.e., [V + PP]), an order not seen in the other seven children. This order was interpreted as an influence from English (Yip & Matthews, 2007) as LTF had been cared for by a Filipina domestic helper full time since birth. LTF's mother spent more time with LTF a year and a half later when she started working from home. Although LTF communicated mostly in Cantonese, she was reported to use "something English-like" with the domestic helper (Lee, 1994). An appreciation of the language context at home and the community at large is therefore necessary for understanding children's language development and interpreting the patterns observed.

3.2 MLU in English and in Cantonese

The one index of grammatical development that has a long history in child language research is mean length of utterance (MLU) in morphemes (Brown, 1973). Studies on English-speaking children reported three key facts about MLU. First, MLU changes predictably with age, as can be seen in studies reporting a strong correlation (e.g., r = .70, .75 and .88) (Blake et al., 1993; Klee et al., 1989; Miller & Chapman, 1981, respectively). Second, MLU discriminates children with developmental language disorder (DLD)[1] from their typically developing age peers (e.g., Rice et al., 2010). Third, MLU correlates strongly with summary measures of grammatical development such as the Index of Syntax Development (r = .92) (Scarborough et al., 1991) and Blake et al.'s (1993) syntactic complexity measure (r = .88).

The evidence for MLU as an index of grammatical development is, however, incomplete for Cantonese. There was one study that examined the relationship between age and MLU using the Cantonese HKU-70X samples (Study 1, Klee et al., 2004). The children were between 2;6 (years;months) and 5;6 years of age, similar to those in the studies cited earlier. A linear relationship with a correlation coefficient of .44, a value that is lower than that reported for English-speaking children, was observed. Evidence from the second study in Klee et al. (2004) indicated that Cantonese-speaking children with DLD had similar MLUs (based on 100 utterance samples) as the younger typically developing children matched on language levels but significantly lower MLUs than their age peers. There has been no report to date, however, that documents whether there is any relationship between MLU and grammatical development in typically developing children or children with DLD. We will examine this relationship after we have established that MLU100 is a valid proxy index of grammatical development in Cantonese using the *Grammatical Analysis of Cantonese Samples* (GACS) (Wong et al., 2021b) in the next section.

3.3 MLU100 as a valid proxy index of grammatical development in Cantonese

In this section, we report on three pieces of evidence from an analysis of conversational samples in the HKU-70X corpus to argue that MLU100 can serve as a proxy index of grammatical development in Cantonese-speaking preschool children. Unlike Klee et al.'s (2004) Study 1 referred to earlier, in which all complete and intelligible utterances in the samples were used, we included only the first 100 utterances in the analysis. The relationship between age and MLU100 was therefore first re-established with the shorter samples. A slightly higher age-MLU100 correlation of .49 (95% CI = .29 – .65) was observed, but the age-MLU100 relationship generally replicated that reported in Klee et al. (2004), as can be seen in the scatterplot presented in Figure 3.1. Since neither age nor MLU100 were normally distributed (Shapiro-Wilk (1, 70) = .931, p = .001), the Spearman's rho was used in the correlation analysis.

As seen in Figure 3.1, data points appear to be more clustered together above than below the relatively flat regression line, despite the fact that there were a few high-performing outliers who did much better than their age peers. Below the regression line, there were children at different ages who had the same low MLU100 (e.g., 1.5), and a few children in the oldest 5;0 and 5;6 groups had MLU100s that were more similar to those of children in the younger age groups. This distribution resulted in the lower age-MLU (Klee et al., 2004) and age-MLU100 reported in this sample of Cantonese-speaking children, when compared to English-speaking children. Klee et al. (2004) attributed this substantial difference in the age-MLU relationship to the features of Cantonese. Another plausible explanation is that some of the conversational samples used for generating the MLUs or MLU100s might not truly reflect the child's actual language ability. Johnston (2001) presented

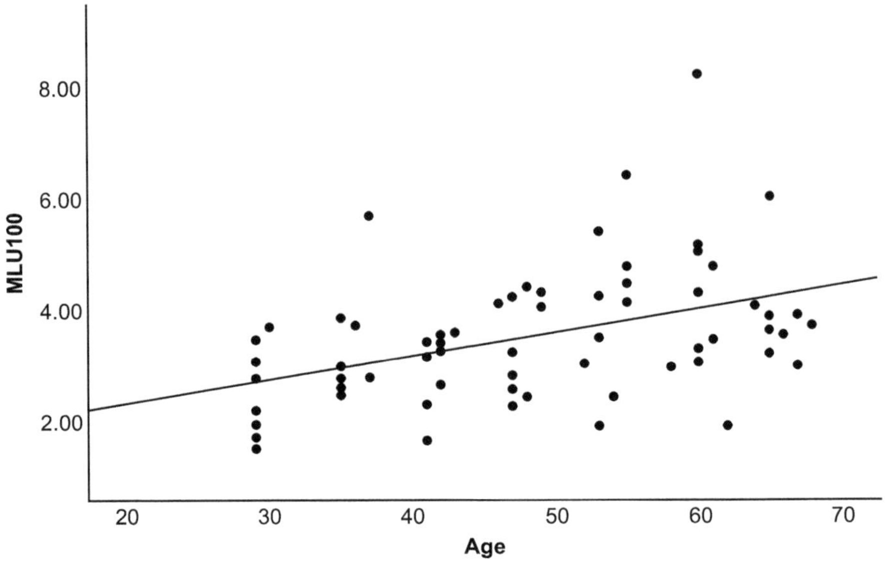

FIGURE 3.1 Scatterplot of age (in months) and MLU100, with the linear regression line, for typically developing Cantonese-speaking children

evidence on the lowering effect of adult discourse features, including yes/no questions and other questions leading to elliptical responses, on children's MLU. This effect was observed in NYW, a 5;7 child who had an MLU100 of 2.97. Seventy-three of his 100 utterances followed a question from the investigator. Not all of his responses to questions were necessarily short; one of them, in fact, contained 15 words. But a majority of his utterances were 1 to 3 words in length, and this probably explains why he had an unexpectedly low MLU100. Given the fact that he could produce a 15-word utterance, it is plausible that the sample might not have been able to tap his actual grammatical capacity. It remains to be seen whether questions from communication partners also explained the unexpectedly low MLU100 in some of the children in the HKU-70X samples. It is clear, however, that samples that are not representative of the children's actual language ability have a larger impact on the age-MLU100 correlation, and the group means of MLU100, when the number of samples in the analysis is small.

Back to MLU100 as a potential proxy index. Klee et al.'s (2004) Study 2 provided the second piece of evidence. As reported in Section 3.2, MLU100 was found to distinguish children with DLD and their typically developing age peers as a group. Here, we present for the first time the third piece of evidence, which was the relationship between MLU100 and grammatical development in typically developing children as measured by the GACS Grand Total score. Figure 3.2 illustrates a strong linear relationship, as reflected in the Spearman rho of .86 ($p < .01$, CI = .78 and .91), which is consistent with what was reported for English-speaking children. Figure 3.3 illustrates how the trends for MLU100 and the GACS Grand

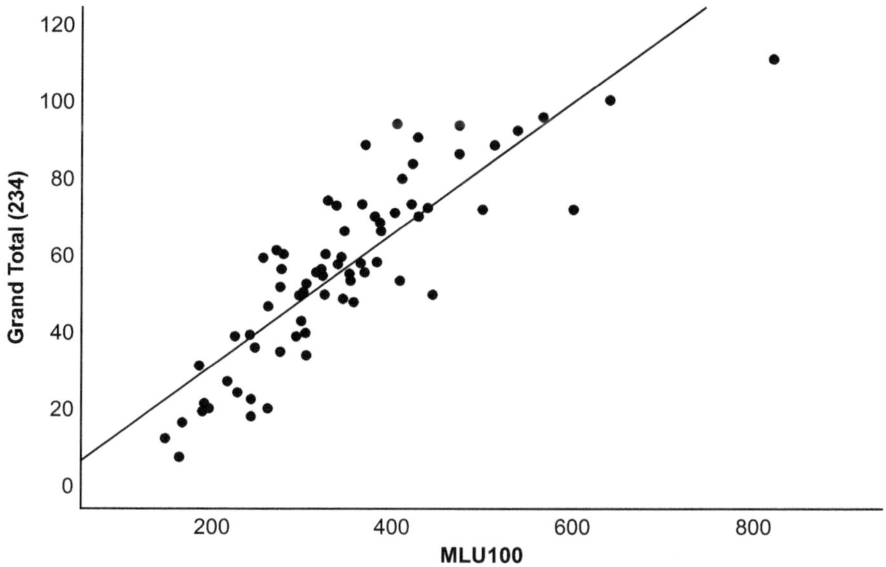

FIGURE 3.2 Scatterplot of GACS Grand Total and MLU100, with the linear regression line, for typically developing Cantonese-speaking children

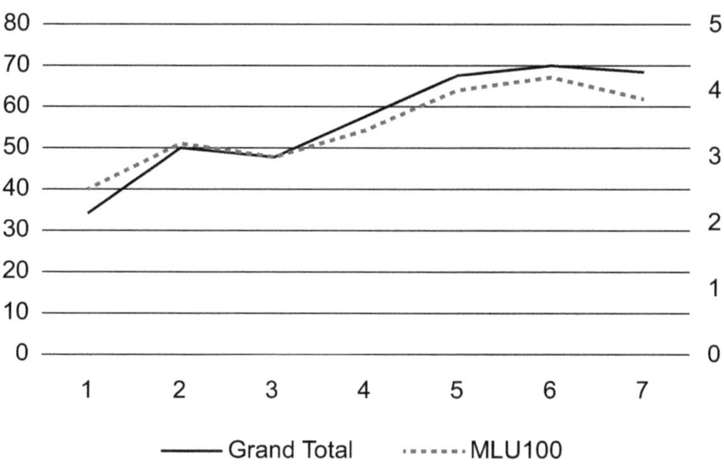

FIGURE 3.3 MLU100 and GACS Grand Total by age group

Total mirrored each other across the age groups. The MLU100 and the GACS Grand Total for the older age group were higher than the immediately younger age group, except between groups 2 and 3 and between groups 6 and 7. To conclude from the three pieces of evidence just presented, MLU100 is a developmentally sensitive proxy index of grammatical development in Cantonese-speaking children between 2;6 and 5;6.

3.4 GACS scores as valid summative measures of grammatical development in Cantonese

Unlike MLU, which is a proxy index, the GACS Grand Total and GACS subscores directly capture children's grammatical knowledge and use. Instead of three, two pieces of evidence are therefore needed to ascertain that GACS scores are valid summative measures of grammatical development. The first is that there is a relationship between age and the scores. This relationship was examined using the cross-sectional Cantonese HKU-70 corpus and longitudinal data from one child in the CANCORP. The second is that the scores discriminate children with and without DLD as a group. We will present these two pieces of evidence in turn.

3.4.1 Relationship between age and GACS scores in cross-sectional samples

Table 3.1 shows summary statistics for age, MLU100, the GACS Grand Total and GACS subscores for each of the seven groups of children and the group as a whole in the HKU-70X corpus. Note that the analysis reported here used an earlier and slightly different version of the GACS (Wong et al., 2021b), in which fewer exemplars for some of the items were included. For example, only two instead of the standard four exemplars were requested for the Other Auxiliaries in the Verb Phrase Expansion section. In the Sentence Structures section, the 到 *dou3* [to be followed by] construction under Sentences with a Preposition Phrase and complex Serial Verb Constructions were not included. In addition, only the standard four exemplars of Clausal Complements were requested. In the Questions section, only two exemplars of the eight types of yes/no questions and the standard four exemplars for *wh* questions were included. So the maximum section scores and the maximum Grand Total were lower in this earlier version than in the version described in Chapter 2.

The third author of Chapter 2 completed scoring for the 70 samples in the HKU-70X corpus, the 45 samples from Wong et al. (2010) and LLY's 20 samples from the CANCORP. To examine inter-rater reliability, 14 samples from the HKU-70X and 10 samples from the Wong et al. (2010) corpus were scored independently by the fourth author. Both scorers contributed to the development of the GACS and received training on the analysis from the first author before scoring the samples. Correlations of their GACS Grand Total scores and GACS subscores were high, with range of .86 to .98.

Now, let's take a look at the correlation between age and the GACS Grand Total and GACS subscores. Table 3.2 presents the correlation matrix. Interestingly, the age and the GACS Grand Total correlation were the same as that between age and MLU100, with Spearman's rho equaled to .49 (95% CI = .29 – .65). The scatterplot in Figure 3.4 shows a clear linear relationship. There was a significant correlation between age and all GACS subscores as well, except for Questions, with a value ranging between .43 and .54.

TABLE 3.1 Sample size, age (mean and range), RDLS-C scores, MLU100, and the GACS Grand Total and subscores (mean and standard deviation) for each group in the Cantonese HKU-70X corpus

		Age (months)		*RDLS-C*		*MLU 100*		*NP (max 28)*		*VP (max 54)*		*Sentences (max 84)*		*Questions (max 20)*		*S. Adv., Conj. & SFP (max 48)*		*Grand Total (max 234)*	
Gp	*n*	*M*	*range*	*M*	*SD*	*M*	*SD*	*M*	*SD*	*M*	*SD*	*M*	*SD*	*M*	*SD*	*M*	*SD*	*M*	*SD*
1	10	29.1	27–30	32.0	7.3	2.5	0.8	2.9	2.1	9.2	6.5	11.1	6.0	3.8	2.2	7.6	4.8	34.7	19.6
2	10	35.5	35–37	46.0	7.7	3.2	1.0	5.1	4.6	12.9	5.8	16.4	7.3	4.9	2.1	11.1	5.9	50.4	22.2
3	10	41.7	41–43	48.0	5.9	3.0	0.6	5.0	2.6	12.0	5.6	15.8	6.4	4.3	2.4	11.0	4.5	48.1	19.3
4	10	47.5	46–49	51.4	5.1	3.4	0.9	4.3	2.0	15.9	6.3	19.0	5.8	6.0	3.0	12.5	4.5	57.7	17.8
5	10	53.8	52–55	56.1	4.1	4.0	1.4	5.2	2.5	18.6	7.9	21.8	8.9	6.9	4.5	14.8	4.9	67.6	27.0
6	10	60.2	58–62	56.9	3.6	4.2	1.8	6.8	3.9	19.3	8.2	22.7	7.2	4.7	4.6	16.3	7.8	70.2	28.4
7	10	65.7	64–68	60.7	2.2	3.9	0.8	7.3	3.0	18.1	4.8	20.6	5.6	5.3	4.2	17.0	3.7	68.6	15.0
Total	70	47.6	27–68	50.2	10.3	3.5	1.2	5.2	3.2	15.1	7.2	18.2	7.5	5.1	3.4	12.9	6.0	56.8	24.2

RDLS: Reynell Developmental Language Scales (Cantonese)-Comprehension, NP: Noun Phrase Expansion, VP = Verb Phrase Expansion, S. Adv.: Sentence Adverbs, Conj.: Conjunctions, SFP: Sentence Final Particles

TABLE 3.2 Correlation matrix of age, MLU100 and the GAS Grand Total and subscores

	Age	*MLU 100*	*NP*	*VP*	*Sentences*	*Questions*	*S. Adv., Conj. & SFPs*	*Grand Total*
Age	1							
MLU	.49**	1						
NP	.43**	.74**	1					
VP	.48**	.77**	.65**	1				
Sentences	.48**	.81**	.71**	.83**	1			
Questions	.10	.55**	.39**	.59**	.49**	1		
S Adv, Conj & SFPs	.54**	.84**	.79**	.82**	.81**	.49**	1	
Grand Total	.49**	.86**	.80**	.93**	.93**	.63**	.91**	1

**Correlation is significant at the 0.01 level (2-tailed)
NP: Noun Phrase Expansion, VP = Verb Phrase Expansion, S. Adv.: Sentence Adverbs, Conj.: Conjunctions, SFP: Sentence Final Particles

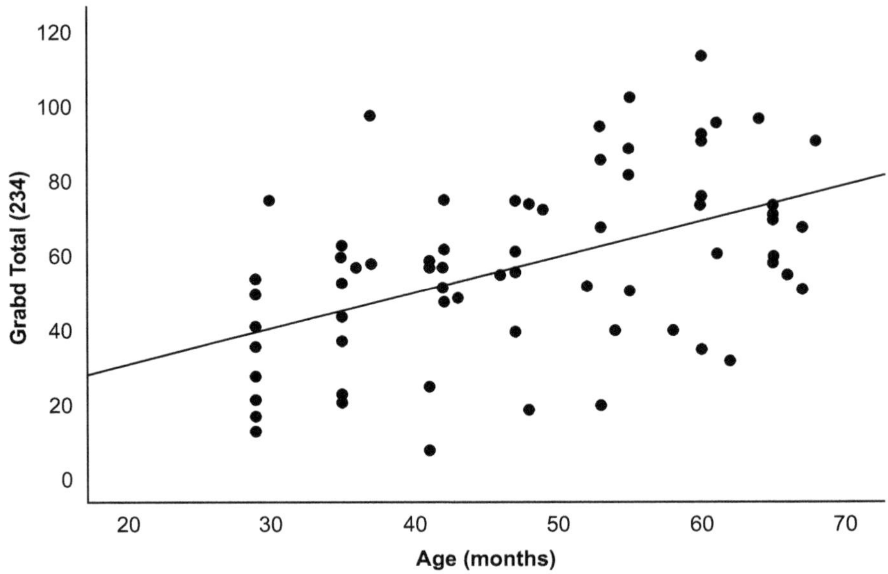

FIGURE 3.4 Scatterplot of age and the GACS Grand Total, with the linear regression line, for typically developing Cantonese-speaking children

To identify converging evidence on the relationship between age and GACS scores, we now turn to the 20-sample data set from LLY in the CANCORP. Table 3.3 shows summary statistics for age, MLU100, the GACS Grand Total and GACS subscores when LLY was between 2;8 and 3;8 years. Table 3.4 presents the

TABLE 3.3 LLY's MLU100, her GACS Grand Total and GACS subscores from her 20 conversation samples collected between 2;8 and 3;8 years

	Age (months)		*MLU 100*		*NP (max 28)*		*VP (max 54)*		*Sentences (max 84)*		*Questions (max 20)*		*S. Adv., Conj. & SFP (max 48)*		*Grand Total (max 234)*	
	M	*range*	*M*	*SD*	*M*	*SD*	*M*	*SD*	*M*	*SD*	*M*	*SD*	*M*	*SD*	*M*	*SD*
LLY	37.6	32–44	3.2	0.7	7.4	3.2	21.8	6.7	25.5	6.2	7.6	3.3	14.6	3.4	76.8	19.5

NP: Noun Phrase Expansion, VP: Verb Phrase Expansion, S. Adv.: Sentence Adverbs, Conj.: Conjunctions, SFP: Sentence Final Particles

TABLE 3.4 Correlation matrix between age, MLU100, the GACS Grand Total and the GACS subscores for data from LLY

	Age	*MLU*	*NP*	*VP*	*Sentences*	*Questions*	*S. Adv., Conj. & SFPs*	*Grand Total*
Age	1							
MLU	.63**	1						
NP	.75**	.67**	1					
VP	.59**	.32	.61**	1				
Sentences	.64**	.58**	.67**	.61**	1			
Questions	.82**	.62**	.84**	.73**	.70**	1		
S. Adv, Conj & SFPs	.89**	.61**	.74**	.62**	.61**	.78**	1	
Grand Total	.82**	.61**	.85**	.86**	.86**	.91**	.83**	1

** Correlation is significant at the 0.01 level (2-tailed).
RDLS: Reynell Developmental Language Scales (Cantonese)-Comprehension, NP: Noun Phrase Expansion, VP: Verb Phrase Expansion, S. Adv.: Sentence Adverbs, Conj.: Conjunctions, SFP: Sentence Final Particles

correlation matrix between age, MLU100, the GACS Grand Total and GACS subscores. The Pearson correlation coefficient for age and the GACS Grand Total was .82 (95% CI = .59 and .93), revealing a strong linear relationship as seen in the scatterplot in Figure 3.5.

There was a correlation between age and all GACS subscores, including the Questions subscore, with values ranging between .59 and .89. These results generally replicated those reported on the HKU-70X corpus earlier in this Section of 3.4.1, except that the correlations were higher in LLY's samples. One obvious

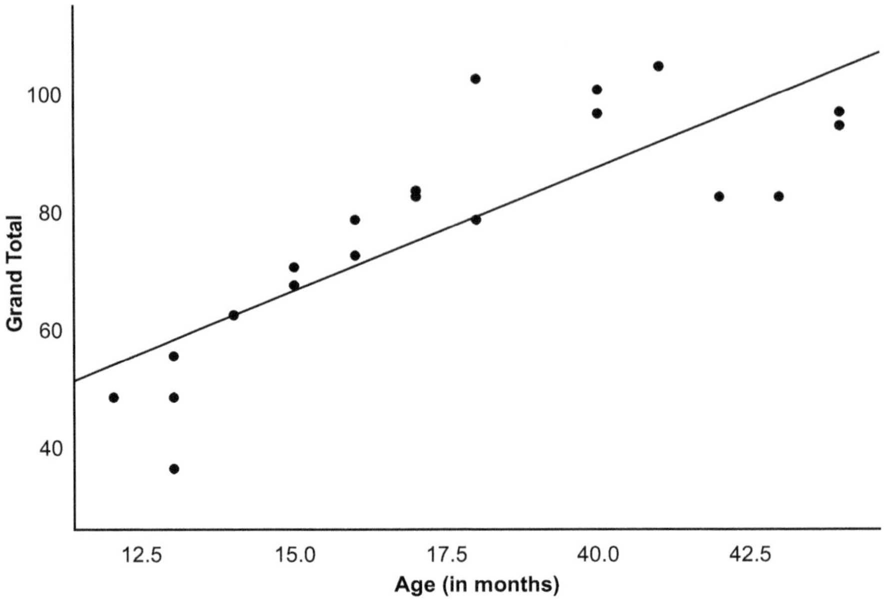

FIGURE 3.5 Scatterplot of age (in months) and GACS Grand Total with linear regression line for LLY

explanation of this difference is that the LLY samples were collected from one single child spanning a much narrower time frame of just 12 months, thus restricting the variabilities across time.

Although this section focuses primarily on the relationship between age and the GACS scores, a result from the correlation analysis of LLY's GACS scores and MLU100s is particularly noteworthy. As is clear from Table 3.4, among all the correlation coefficients, the only one that is not statistically significant is between the GACS Verb Phrase Expansion subscore and MLU100. Figure 3.6 illustrates a curvilinear relationship, which was marked by a clear drop in Verb Phrase Expansion when MLU100 was between 4 and 4.5. For these four highest MLU100s, three had a corresponding score in Verb Phrase Expansion that actually fell below the mean.

How did LLY achieve the high MLU100s without much Verb Phrase Expansion? Table 3.5 gives the corresponding GACS subscores for LLY's four data points where MLU100 was higher than 4. One possible answer was through other means, particularly the use of longer and complex Sentence Structures as well as different Sentence Adverbs, Conjunctions and Sentence Final Particles. When Table 3.5 is examined in relation to Table 3.3, it is clear that in all four data points where MLU100 was higher than 4, LLY scored higher than the mean in these two sections on the GACS.

While this answer makes sense, it is important to note that not all children showed a drop in Verb Phrase Expansion when their MLU100 was 4 or above. As

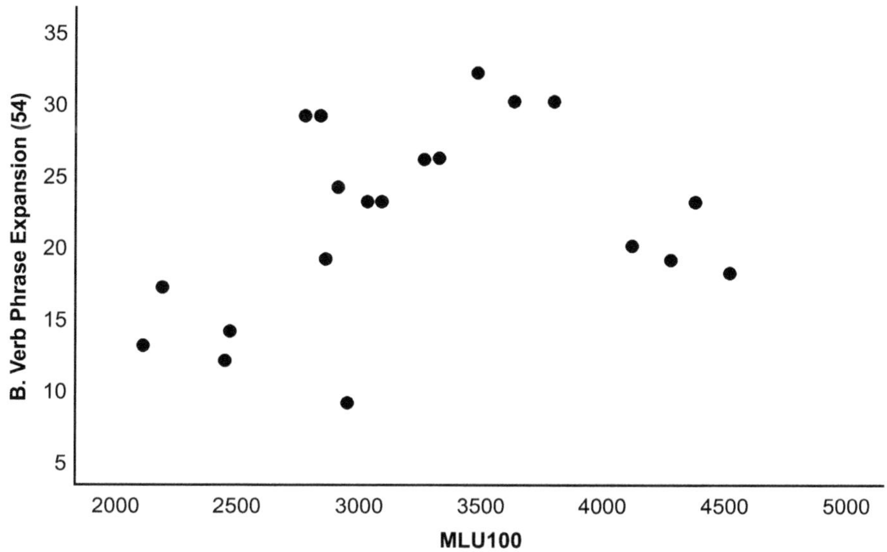

FIGURE 3.6 Scatterplot of MLU100s and GACS Verb Phrase Expansion subscores for LLY

TABLE 3.5 GACS subscores for the four data points where LLY's MLU100 is higher than 4

	Age (months)	*MLU100*	*NP (max 28)*	*VP (max 54)*	*Sentences (max 84)*	*Questions (max 20)*	*S. Adv, Conj. & SFP (max 48)*	*Grand Total (max 234)*
LLY30130	38	4.12	7	20	27	7	17	78
LLY30616	43	4.28	7	19	29	9	18	82
LLY30213	38	4.38	12	23	41	10	16	102
LLY30520	42	4.52	13	18	22	12	17	82

NP: Noun Phrase Expansion, VP: Verb Phrase Expansion, S. Adv.: Sentence Adverbs, Conj.: Conjunctions, SFP: Sentence Final Particles

seen in Figure 3.7, while a few children in the cross-sectional HKU-70X samples with MLU100 higher than 4 received a Verb Phrase Expansion subscore that was lower than children with a lower MLU100, many children scored high on both MLU100 and Verb Phrase Expansion. This suggests that there did not have to be a trade-off between Verb Phrase Expansion and other aspects of grammar that contributed to children's increase in mean utterance length. In fact, the two children with MLU100 above 6 in the HKU-70X samples had not only a very high score on Verb Phrase Expansion but also a score that was above the mean for their groups on the other sections, except Questions. Therefore, what we observed in LLY was

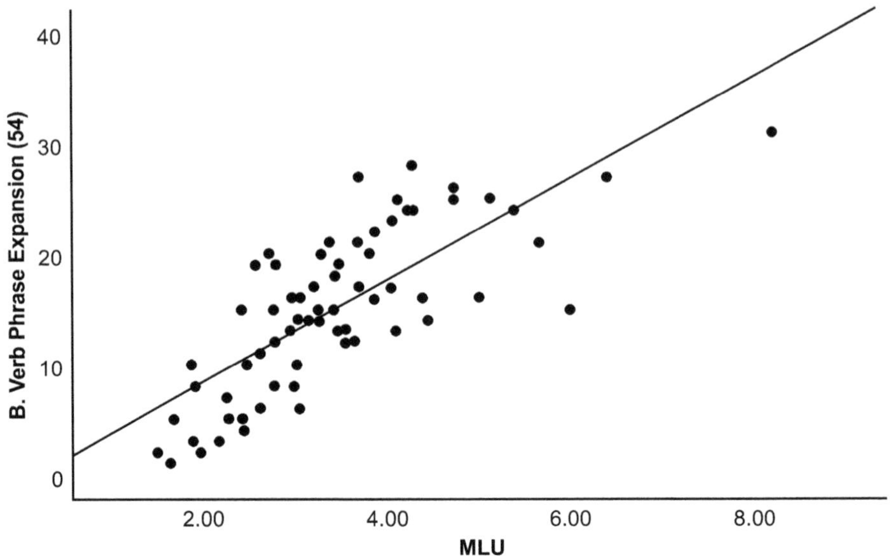

FIGURE 3.7 Scatterplot of MLU100s and the GACS Verb Phrase Expansion, with the linear regression line, for typically developing Cantonese-speaking children

likely a feature of individual differences in the grammatical options children took to elaborate their meanings during a particular phase of language development.

3.4.2 Differences between children with and without DLD in GACS scores

In this section, we examine differences between children with and without DLD on GACS scores using the 45 samples reported in Wong et al. (2010). The samples came from three groups of children: 15 five-year-old children with DLD (DLD group), 15 typically developing age peers (O-TD group), and 15 three-year-old typically developing children matched on the comprehension score of the Reynell Developmental Language Scale-Cantonese (Reynell & Huntley, 1987) (Y-TD group). Table 3.6 shows summary statistics for age, MLU100, the GACS Grand Total and GACS subscores for each of the three groups of children and the groups as a whole. Scores for each of the variables were normally distributed by age group, as indicated by $p > .05$ in the Shapiro Wilk test, except for the Y-TD group's Sentence Structures subscores and the DLD group's Sentence Adverbs, Conjunctions and Sentence Final Particles subscores.

Univariate ANOVA was used to examine group differences in each of the variables. Homogeneity of variances was confirmed for all variables, except age, using the Levene's test. Table 3.7 summarizes the results of the analyses. There were statistically significant differences among groups in most variables of interest, including MLU100, Noun Phrase Expansion, Verb Phrase Expansion, Sentence

TABLE 3.6 Summary statistics for age, MLU100, GACS Grand Total and GACS subscores for 45 children in three groups

		Age (months)		*RDLS-C*		*MLU 100*		*NP (max 28)*		*VP (max 54)*		*Sentences (max 84)*		*Questions (max 20)*		*S. Adv, Conj. & SFP (max 48)*		*Grand Total (max 234)*	
Gp	*n*	*M*	*range*	*M*	*SD*	*M*	*SD*	*M*	*SD*	*M*	*SD*	*M*	*SD*	*M*	*SD*	*M*	*SD*	*M*	*SD*
O-TD	15	60.5	49–81	56.5	2.7	4.5	0.8	6.1	2.2	20.7	3.9	20.3	4.7	6.9	3.1	16.1	3.3	134.1	19.8
Y-TD	15	37.7	35–42	41.5	5.6	3.8	0.6	4.3	1.5	15.8	3.8	18.3	6.0	5.0	3.4	11.1	3.3	104.8	27.2
DLD	15	60.7	50–80	43.6	6.7	3.8	0.7	5.7	1.6	15.1	4.2	15.7	4.8	5.6	2.4	11.5	3.3	101.6	21.6
Total	45	53.0	35–81	47.2	8.5	4.0	0.8	5.4	1.9	17.2	4.6	18.1	5.4	5.8	3.0	12.9	3.9	113.5	26.9

DLD: children with developmental language disorder, O-TD: same age typically developing peers, Y-TD: younger typically developing controls, RDLS: Reynell Developmental Language Scales (Cantonese)-Comprehension, NP: Noun Phrase Expansion, VP: Verb Phrase Expansion, S. Adv.: Sentence Adverbs, Conj.: Conjunctions, SFP: Sentence Final Particles

TABLE 3.7 Summary of results from univariate ANOVA analyses on the background variables and GACS scores of the 45 children

Variable	*F (2,42)*	*p*	*Partial* η^2	*90% CIs*	*O-TD > Y-TD*	*O-TD > DLD*	*DLD > Y-TD*
Age	63.81	.000	.75	.62–.81	★		★
RDLS-C	35.43	.000	.63	.45–.71	★	★	
MLU100	5.10	.010	.20	.03–.34	★	★	
NP	4.29	.020	.17	.02–.31	★		
VP	8.73	.001	.29	.10–.43	★	★	
Sentences	2.96	.063	.12	.00–.26			
Questions	1.65	.205	.07	.00–.19			
S. Adv., Conj., SFP	10.50	.000	.33	.13–.47	★	★	
Grand Total	9.03	.001	.30	.10–.44	★	★	

DLD: children with developmental language disorder, O-TD: same age typically developing peers, Y-TD: younger typically developing controls, RDLS-C (Reynell Developmental Language Scales (Cantonese)-Comprehension, NP: Noun Phrase Expansion, VP: Verb Phrase Expansion, S. Adv.: Sentence Adverbs, Conj.: Conjunctions, SFP: Sentence Final Particles

Adverbs, Conjunctions, Sentence Final Particles and the GACS Grand Total. The magnitude of the effect size suggested that these group differences were important, despite the confidence intervals being rather wide for some variables, plausibly a result of small sample size. Specifically, except for Noun Phrase Expansion, the other variables showed the same expected pattern of differences (O-TD > Y-TD, O-TD > DLD, Y-TD ~ DLD).

Although group differences for Sentences were not statistically significant, a moderate-to-large effect size suggested that a larger sample size might mitigate the large variabilities within groups, leading to a different result. The absence of group differences for Questions was not unexpected, given their low incidence and variable use in conversation, from which the samples were collected. In sum, the univariate analyses provided the evidence that GACS Grand Total and several GACS subscores discriminated children with and without DLD.

Given evidence that GACS scores are developmentally sensitive and can discriminate children with and without DLD, we conclude that GACS scores can be considered valid summative measures of grammatical development in Cantonese-speaking preschool children.

3.5 MLU100 vs. GACS scores as valid measures of grammatical development

So far, we have established that both MLU100 and GACS scores are valid measures of grammatical development in Cantonese-speaking preschool children. The two measures are, however, rather different in nature. As a measure of mean utterance length, MLU100 is only a proxy index of a child's knowledge of grammar. Calculated on the basis of the actual grammatical forms and structures used by the child, GACS scores are direct summative measures of a child's grammar. How do we choose which one to use? It depends on our goal: that is, why we do what we do.

MLU100 is easy to generate, especially if the language samples have been formatted in ways that allow automatic reading and analysis by commercial programs like Systematic Analysis of Language Transcripts (Salt, 2021) or free programs like those provided in the Child Language Data Exchange System (CHILDES, MacWhinney, 2000). MLU100 is therefore a quick and easy index to document change in a child's grammar quantitatively over time and to make comparisons between children. There are, however, two caveats for the use of MLU100. First, MLU100 depends on an unambiguous definition of word and utterance, as well as clear operational guidelines on utterance segmentation. Utterance segmentation for Cantonese narrative samples was reported to be low in inter-rater reliability (To et al., 2010). It is likely that inter-rater reliability is higher for Cantonese conversational samples, given that a speaking turn from the communication partner can provide a natural cue for the end of the speaker's utterance. This is especially true when the samples are collected from well-trained conversational partners with strong clinical discourse skills. Nevertheless, inter-rater reliability in utterance segmentation has not been examined or reported in any of the four corpora of conversational samples of Cantonese-speaking preschool children reported in Table 2.1 in Chapter 2.

Second, MLU100 provides no information on what specific grammatical knowledge the child has at his or her disposal. Hence, the same MLU100 value from two different conversational samples may reflect different profiles across aspects of grammar, as can be inferred from an illustration using these two utterances from a 3;5 child.

[A] 姐姐攞功課做喇。

ze4ze1	*lo2*	*gung1fo3*	*zou6*	*laa3*
older-sister	take	homework	do	SFP

(The older sister takes out her homework to do.)

[B] 我行吓街咋！

ngo5	*haang4*	*haa5*	*gaai1*	*zaa3*
I	walk	ASP	street	SFP

(I am just going for a walk!)

[A] has seven syllables, and [B] has five. But since both 姐姐 *ze4ze1* [older-sister] and 功課 *gung1fo3* [homework] in [A] are bi-syllabic words, [A] and [B] actually both contain five words, with the last one being a Sentence Final Particle. Despite the same number of words, [A] and [B] display very different grammatical characteristics. [A] contains a Serial Verb Construction formed by the verbs

攞 *lo2* [take] and 做 *zou6* [do], and neither of them is modified. On the other hand, [B] contains just one verb, but the verb 行 *haang4* [walk] is modified by the aspect marker 吓 *haa5*.

GACS scores can be used to document quantitative change in a child's grammar over time and to make comparisons between children in the same way MLU100 does. Because GACS scores are generated from a qualitative analysis of the language sample, speech-language therapists can develop a thorough understanding of the specific forms and structures (e.g., Complements of the verb, Prepositional Phrases or Serial Verb Constructions) that the child does not use or uses with errors. As a result, the analysis can help speech-language therapists identify targets for further probing and/or intervention (Owens et al., 2018). Having said that, the downsides to GACS scores versus MLU100 are the amount of time they take and the necessary expertise required for the qualitative grammatical analysis. These barriers can be overcome once one is familiar with the GACS framework after practice and when technology is available to automate part of the analysis process. For the latter, a platform like Language Explorer (Language Explorer, 2021) can be developed for use with Cantonese-speaking children in the future.

Ultimately, the choice between MLU100 and GACS scores depends on the goal of the users. One important point to note is that meaningful use of either of these measures, first and foremost, depends on the availability of a representative conversational sample. Factors that affect the representativeness of conversational samples include sample length, conversational topics, language sampling contexts and materials (Voniati et al., 2021). It is beyond the scope of this chapter to discuss best practice in language sampling. For practical suggestions, please refer to Nippold (2021).

3.6 A qualitative overview of grammatical development in Cantonese-speaking children by age group

In previous sections, we reported on grammatical development in Cantonese-speaking children using quantitative measures. In this and the next section, we provide a qualitative overview of grammatical development using the GACS framework first by age group and then by individual.

Not all aspects of grammar are learned at the same time. The ones that are conceptually and formally more complex are learned later than the simpler ones (Clark, 2003). These two sources of complexity determine the general order of grammatical development observed in a majority of children. Differences in the quality and quantity of language input, personal interests and learning styles and learning capacity, however, can moderate this general order in individual children.

For the purpose of curriculum development and screening children at risk for language difficulties, early childhood educators and speech-language therapists often refer to the age and order of development of various aspects of language. Summarized on the basis of experience rather than research evidence, many Cantonese language-development milestone charts that are easily accessible only cover very general aspects of development within a very wide age range (Heep Hong Society, 1995; Education Bureau, 2008). There is a need for an objective investigation of the development of Cantonese through a more systematic analysis of language samples using a well-described framework.

In this section, we report on the order and age of emergence and productive use of each aspect of grammar included in the same earlier version of the GACS framework (Wong et al., 2021b) used in the quantitative analysis reported in Section 3.4. The conversational samples came again from the HKU-70X corpus. Recall that two-to-five-year-old children sampled in the HKU-70X corpus fell into seven groups, six months apart. The age of the children in each group fell within a narrow range of two months. Recall that we scored each aspect of grammar – that is, each item in the GACS framework – by type but not by token. The age of emergence (AE) of an item was defined as the age at which seven or more children received a score of 1 or more. The age of productive use (AP) was defined as the age at which eight or more children received a score of 2 or more.

We summarize here the findings on the AE and the AP for each item following the organization of the GACS framework section by section. Of all the different types of Noun Phrase Expansion, Classifiers emerged the earliest at 2;6 and were used productively at 3;0. This report of early emergence is consistent with earlier studies (Szeto, 1996). Adjectival Modifiers and Possessive Constructions emerged at five years of age, later than expected. Other elements that elaborate the meaning of Noun Phrases, including Nominal Modifiers, Locative Modifiers, Prepositional Modifiers and Relative Clauses, did not meet the criteria for emergence or productive use. One plausible explanation is that the focus on the here-and-now objects and events did not obligate the use of these structures during conversations on a standard toy set with dolls around the bathing routine.

There was much going on in Verb Phrase Expansion during the preschool period. Negation Adverbs and Directional Particles emerged early at 2;6, although none of them met the criteria of productive use. The result on Negation Adverbs was consistent with Tam and Stokes's (2001) report of their analysis of the eight children in the CANCORP. These eight children used the Negation Adverb 唔 *m4* [not] the most often, followed by 冇 *mou5* [not have] and 未 *mei6* [not yet]. Of note is the fact that Directional Particles were the first Verbal Particles to emerge. Modal Auxiliaries, Degree Adverbs, Aspect Markers and Resultative Particles all emerged at 3;0. Modal Auxiliaries and Resultative Particles were used productively at 4;0, slightly earlier than Aspect Markers at 4;6. Other Particles emerged at 3;6, later than Resultative Particles and Aspect Markers. Manner Adverbs emerged later at 5;6.

Regarding Sentence Structures, Verb-Object Sentences emerged and were used productively early at 2;6. Subject-Verb Sentences also emerged at 2;6 but reached productive use one year later at 3;6. Canonical Subject-Verb-Object Sentences emerged and were used productively at 3. In adult Cantonese, the object or the subject can be dropped where it has been established as the topic of the discourse or where the reference is clear from the context (Matthews & Yip, 2011). Data from the CANCORP (Man, 1996) revealed that both subject drop and object drop were substantially more prevalent in young Cantonese-speaking children than what was reported in their English-speaking peers and that subject drop (Verb-Object Sentences) was more common than object drop (Subject-Verb Sentences). For example, between the months of 2;05 and 2,07/2;08, one child had a subject group rate of 85% and an object drop rate of 55% while the other child had a subject drop rate of 78% and an object drop rate of 49%. The fact that Verb-Object Sentences reached the level of productive use earlier than Subject-Verb Sentences in this sample of children was consistent with results from Man (1996).

Of special note is that Serial Verb Constructions, which emerged at the same time as Subject-Verb-Object sentences, reached the level of productive use at 4;6. This provides additional evidence for the early and productive use of Serial Verb Constructions in the preschool years (Fung, 2011; Tse et al., 2002). Pivotal constructions emerged at 5;0, later than Serial Verb Constructions, as Pivotal Constructions are syntactically more complex despite their similarities in surface structure. Subject-Adjective Sentences emerged at 4;0, and Clausal Complements emerged at 4;6. Complex Sentences without Explicit Conjunctions did not reach the criteria of emergence or productive use in this sample of children.

Questions were not observed much in the children in the HKU-70X corpus, probably an effect of conversational topics and the length of the language samples. Of all question types, only one type of yes/no questions – Particle Questions – and *wh* questions reached the criteria of emergence. *Wh* questions showed productive use at 4;0. Wong and Ingram (2003) completed an analysis of children's questions in the CANCORP. Of the three types, particle/intonation questions were reported as being acquired first, followed by *wh* questions and then A-not-A questions. Note that not all *wh* questions were acquired before A-not-A questions. The order of acquisition of the *wh* questions was what > where, why > who, how, although individual variability in this general order was observed.

The last section in the GACS framework is a collection of three sets of items, including Sentence Adverbs, Conjunctions and Sentence Final Particles. Of note is that Sentence Final Particles emerged and were used productively at 2;6 and plausibly earlier, as observed in Lee et al. (1996). Regarding Sentence Adverbs, Temporal Adverbs emerged early at 3;0 and were used productively at 4;0 while Scope Adverbs and Frequency Adverbs emerged later at 4;0 and at 4;6, respectively. Regarding Conjunctions, Temporal Conjunctions were the first ones to emerge at 4;6, followed by Concession Conjunctions at 5;6. Causal Conjunctions, however, did not meet the criteria of either emergence or productive use. In English-speaking children, Temporal and Causal Conjunctions appear at about the same time (around the age of three), with the latter being slightly earlier (Clark, 2003). The same proximity of development of the Temporal and Causal conjunctions was not observed in this sample of Cantonese-speaking children. One plausible explanation is that the play-based conversational samples in the HKU-70X did not provide many opportunities for the use of Causal Conjunctions.

TABLE 3.8 Items that meet the criteria for age of emergence (AE) for each age group across sections in the GACS framework

	MLU		*GACS Grand Total*						
Age	*M*	*SD*	*M*	*SD*	*NP Expansion*	*VP Expansion*	*Sentence Structures*	*Questions*	*Sentence Adverbs, Sentence Final Particles*
2;6	2.5	0.8	34.7	19.6	Cl	NegAdv; DirPrt	VO; SV	Prt-Q; Wh-Q	SFP
3;0	3.2	1.0	50.4	22.2		ModAux; DegAdv; Asp; ResPrt	SVO; SVC		TempAdv
3;6	3.0	0.6	48.1	19.3		OthPrt			
4;0	3.4	0.9	57.7	17.8			SA		SocAdv
4;6	4.0	1.4	67.6	27.0			CC		FreAdv; TempConj
5;0	4.2	1.8	70.2	28.4	AdjMod; Poss		PC		
5;6	3.9	0.8	68.6	15.0		ManAdv			ConcConj

Table 3.8 and Table 3.9 summarize the items that met the criteria for AE and AP, respectively, for each age group across sections in the GACS framework. This summary reveals three interesting facts that were not reported in previous paragraphs focusing on individual sections of the GACS. First, from the earliest age, children developed phrasal and clausal elements in parallel. Second, Sentence Final Particles emerged and were used productively before the canonical sentences and plausibly before combinations of content words as these particles can follow a single noun, as in 車呀！ *ce1 aa3* 'car SFP' [(That's) a car!]. Third, Serial Verb Constructions emerged at the same time as Resultative Particles. This finding was generally consistent with Fung's (2011) report of the CANCORP data that two-verb contiguous Serial Verb Constructions emerged about two months earlier than two-verb non-contiguous Serial Verb Constructions. In her study, two-verb contiguous Serial Verb Constructions included the use of a verb immediately followed by a Directional Particle or a Resultative Particle. Differences in the criteria of emergence in this analysis and in Fung's (2011) study and differences in how spread out in age the children sampled were in the two language sample corpora (cf: Table 2.1) could explain this small discrepancy in findings.

We close this section with three caveats on our qualitative description of the general orders of grammatical development in Cantonese-speaking preschool children. First, the orders were the results of arbitrary, albeit objective, criteria of emergence and productive use. The orders could be different if the number of

TABLE 3.9 Items that meet the criteria for age of productive use (AP) for each age group across sections in the GACS framework

	MLU		*GACS Grand Total*						
Age	*M*	*SD*	*M*	*SD*	*NP Expansion*	*VP Expansion*	*Sentence Structures*	*Questions*	*Sentence Adverbs, Conjunctions, Sentence Final Particles*
2;6	2.5	0.8	34.7	19.6			VO		SFP
3;0	3.2	1.0	50.4	22.2	Cl		SVO		
3;6	3.0	0.6	48.1	19.3			SV		
4;0	3.4	0.9	57.7	17.8		ModAux; ResPrt		Wh-Q	TempAdv
4;6	4.0	1.4	67.6	27.0		Asp	SVC		
5;0	4.2	1.8	70.2	28.4					
5;6	3.9	0.8	68.6	15.0					

TABLE 3.10 Initials, ages, MLU100, GACS Grand Totals and GACS scores of the ten children from HKU-70X

	Child	*Group*	*Age*	*MLU100*	*GACS Grand Total*	*NP (28)#*	*VP (54)*	*SS (84)*	*Q (20)*	*SA, C, SFP (48)*
#1	LWL20520*	1	29	1.49	12	2	2	5	2	1
#2	FYS20527	1	29	2.17	27	5	3	7	5	7
#3	LCK21119	2	35	2.61	20	1	6	7	5	1
#4	CPY30516	3	41	3.14	56	5	14	21	3	13
#5	LHC40527	5	53	3.47	67	5	19	22	6	15
#6	CKK50015	6	60	4.27	92	8	28	28	9	19
#7	HKK50121	6	61	4.73	93	8	26	22	14	23
#8	LJK50005	6	60	5.13	90	12	25	29	4	20
#9	ST40701	5	55	6.4	98	10	23	36	10	19
#10	CWC50010	6	60	8.2	113	14	31	36	3	29

* The numbers indicate the age of the child in years, months and days (20520 = 2 years 5 months and 20 days,
# The number in brackets indicate maximum scores for the section,
NP = Noun Phrase Expansion, VP = Verb Phrase Expansion, SS = Sentence Structures, Q = Questions, SA = Sentence Adverbs, C = Conjunctions, SFP = Sentence Final Particles

TABLE 3.11 A summary of the items observed in the sample of ten children across sections in the GACS framework

	Child	*GACS Grand Total*	*MLU 100*	*Noun Phrase Expansion*	*Verb Phrase Expansion*	*Sentence Structures*	*Questions*	*Sentence Adverbs, Conjunctions, Sentence Final Particles*	*Others*
1	LWL20520	12	1.49	**CL***	**NegAdv**	**VO** **SVC** **SA** **Loc Comp-PP** **Comp A**	**Wh-Q**: **What, Who**	**SFP**	**Focus verb**
2	FYS20527	27	2.17	CL			**Exi Q** **Cop Q**	SFP **Temp Conj:** go2zan6 **Temp Adv**: zung6, tau4sin1	Focus verb; **Extended ditransitive construction**
3	LCK21119	20	2.61	CL			**Wh-Q: Where** **Prt Q**	SFP	Focus verb; **Wh-Q: What for;** **Topic Comment**
4	CPY30516	56	3.14	CL **Adj Mod**	**Mod Aux** **Oth Prt** **Deg Adv**	**CS-Conj (temp)** **S PP bei2**		SFP Temp Conj: go2zan4 **S Adv**: dou1	**Right Dislocation;** **Temporal sequences marked by jyun4**
5	LHC40527	67	3.47		**ASP** Deg Adv Neg Adv **Res Prt** **Dir Prt**	**C-SVC** **CC**		SFP **Coor Conj**: ding6hai6 Temp Conj: zau6 (+ jyun4)	**SA with S being a SVO** **First-person imperative**

(*Continued*)

TABLE 3.11 (Continued)

	Child	*GACS Grand Total*	*MLU 100*	*Noun Phrase Expansion*	*Verb Phrase Expansion*	*Sentence Structures*	*Questions*	*Sentence Adverbs, Conjunctions, Sentence Final Particles*	*Others*
6	CKK50015	92	4.27	CL	ASP Res Prt Neg Adv Dir Prt Mod Aux	C-SVC SVC		SFP Temp Conj (3 clauses): zau6 Temp Conj: zi1hau6 Fre Adv	Extended ditransitive construction
7	HKK50121	93	4.73	CL	Mod Aux Neg Adv Other Prt Dir Prt ASP	**Top** **S PP tung4** **Loc Comp-Loc**		SFP Temp Conj: go2si4 +/-zau6 **Conc Conj**: daan6hai6, bat1gwo3 **Caus Conj**: jan1wai6 **Freq Adv**	**Gapless noun modifying clausal construction;** Focus Marker
8	LJK50005	90	5.13	CL	Dir Prt Res Prt Neg Adv Mod Aux	**PC**		SFP Temp Conj: jin4hau6	First-person imperative; **Second-person imperative;** Topic Comment
9	ST40701	98	6.4	CL **Poss**	**Pot Prt** Dir Prt ASP	SA PC CS-Conj: causal	**A-not-A Q: rhetorical**	SFP **Cond Conj**: (jyu4gwo2) + zau6	**Indirect speech**
10	CWC50010	113	8.2	CL	ASP Res Prt Neg Adv Mod Aux Oth VPrt	C-SVC		SFP Conc Conj: bat1gwo3 Temp Conj: sin1; jin4zi1hau6	

* Refer to the description of the GACS framework in Chapter 2 for the short form used in this table. The items are bolded when they first appeared in this sample of children.

children receiving a certain score in the criteria of emergence and productive use were changed. Second, while the orders we reported here, both within and across the sections in the GACS framework, are consistent with the literature, there are still gaps in our knowledge, especially with regard to Noun Phrase Expansion and Questions. It might be useful to examine the development of Noun Phrase Expansion using language samples collected from a slightly more structured sampling procedure or a story retelling task to complement our findings here. Third, relatively few items were identified as emerging or reaching a productive level in the older age groups from 3;6 on. Given observations reported earlier, it will be necessary to collect supplementary samples using the same play routine for children in this age range, with careful attention to the communicative partners' use of questions and other discourse skills, to ascertain our findings.

While the orders reported here needs to be replicated, we have demonstrated the use of a research methodology for summarizing developmental information obtained from analyses of language samples using the GACS framework. This summary will provide the foundation for future investigation and observation by child language researchers, speech-language therapists and early childhood educators.

3.7 A qualitative overview of grammatical development by individual children

There is much individual variability in language development (Bates et al., 1995). Evidence from the early days of child language research already suggests that the grammar of children at the same age can vary extensively in structural complexity (Brown, 1973). Why is this so? Language development is not driven by a biological clock, where grammatical forms and structures appear at set times for every child. What the child learns is moderated by both child-internal and child-external factors. The internal factors include the child's conceptual and social skills, cognitive capacity, current knowledge of grammar and communication needs. The external factors include the quality and quantity of language input and the number of languages in the ambient environment.

In this section, instead of milestones, we turn to describing the trajectory of grammatical development through a closer look at the profiles of individual children. Specifically, we ask: What kind of grammatical forms and structures in the GACS framework can we see as children produce longer sentences? We answer this question by examining the grammar of some of the three to five longest non-imitative sentences from ten children with a range of MLU100 in the Cantonese HKU-70X samples. One reason that these children were chosen on the basis MLU100 is because MLU100 correlates strongly with GACS Grand Total, a valid summative measure of grammatical development in Cantonese-speaking children. The other reason is that the longest utterances could be automatically extracted from the samples that were in CHAT format. Table 3.10 gives the initials, ages, MLU100, GACS Grand Totals and GACS scores of the children selected for the analysis.

As is clear from Table 3.12, the rank order of MLU100 of the ten children generally paralleled that of the GACS Grand Total. There are two exceptions to this observation. LCK scored lower in the GACS Grand Total than FYS, despite a higher MLU100. CKK and LJK had very similar GACS Grand Total scores despite the fact that they had a .86 difference in MLU100.

This was not unexpected given an imperfect, albeit very high correlation between MLU100 and GACS Grand Totals as reported in Section 3.3. One might notice that the rank order of the age of the children was also not very well aligned with their MLU100 or GACS Grand Totals. There was also only a mild-to-moderate correlation between age and these two measures of language development in this HKU-70X sample of children. In the remainder of this section, we describe the grammar of some of the three to five longest utterances of ten children.

#1 LWL20520 (MLU100 = 1.49; GACS Grand Total = 12)

[1] 毛巾
mou4gan1
Towel
(towel)

[2] 洗
sai2
wash
(wash)

[3] 好呀。
hou2 aa3
good SFP
(Yes, okay.)
(That's good.)

[4] 唔抹。
m4 maat3
not wipe
((I) am not wiping (it).)

[5] 係腳仔。
hai6 goek3zai2
be foot-little
((It) is a foot.)

[6]* 俾。
bei2
give
((I) give (you this).)

[7] 食呢個。
sik6 nei1 go3
eat this CL
((I) eat this one.)

[8] 咩嚟 ？
me1 lei4 gaa3
what SFP SFP
(What's (this)?)

[9] 係姐姐幫我着!
hai6 ze4ze1 bong1 ngo5 zoek3 gaa3
be older-sister help I wear SFP
((It) is my older sister who helped me wear (this)!)

[10] 邊個有綠色？
bin1go3 jau5 luk6 sik1
who have green color
(Who has a green (sticker)?)

[11] 黏喺呢度。
nim4 hai2 nei1dou6
stick at here
(Stick (it) here.)

[12] 呢件靚啲。

ni1 gin6 leng3 di1
this CL pretty a-bit
(This one is prettier.)

For LWL20520, the child with the lowest MLU100, we include some of his shortest sentences to illustrate language features in children at an earlier developing phase. The one- to two-word sentences illustrated in [1]–[6] were responses to Questions of several different types. [2] and [4] were affirmative and negative responses to the A-not-A Questions [2a] and [4a] respectively. LWL's responses to the two questions were syntactically and pragmatically appropriate in the discourse context. Sentence [6], however, was not an appropriate response to the Particle Question [6a]. The isolated use of verbs as in [6] could only be appropriate as an imperative in adult-child interactions or a response to A-not-A Questions. An appropriate answer to [6a] would be a yes or no response, like 好呀 *hou2 aa3* 'good SFP' [Yes, okay] or 唔好 *m4hou2* 'not-good' [No, not okay].

[2a] *沖涼洗唔洗頭呀BB，洗唔洗呀？*
cung1loeng4 sai2-m4-sai2 tau4 aa3 bi4bi1, sai2-m4-sai2 aa3
take-a-shower wash-not-wash head SFP baby, wash-not-wash SFP
(Baby, do (you) wash your hair in your shower?)
[4a] *我哋攞塊布同佢抹抹喎，你抹唔抹呀？*
ngo5dei6 lo2 faai3 bou3 tung4 keoi5 maat3-maat3 wo3, nei5 maat3-m4-maat3 aa3
we take CL cloth help s/he wipe(-wipe) SPF, you wipe-not-wipe SFP
(We use a cloth to help wipe him/her. Do you wipe him/her too?)
[6a] *我哋又搽喎，你俾啲我吖？*
ngo5dei6 jau6 caa4 wo3, nei5 bei2 di1 ngo5 aa1?
we also put-on SFP, you give some I SFP
(We also put (some soap) on. Could you give me some?)

Sentence [3], [4], [5] and [7] all contained two words. In [3], the last word was a Sentence Final Particle. This two-word combination is commonly used to indicate agreement to a suggestion. [4] involved a Negation Adverb *唔 m4* [not]. Both [5] and [7] were Verb-Object combinations, but the former included a copula verb *係 hai6* [be] and the latter a lexical verb *食 sik6* [eat]. LWL asked a *what* question in [8], using a prefabricated structure that sometimes is preceded by the phrase *呢個 nei1 go3* 'this CL' [this]. This form of *what* question is similar to what is commonly seen in English-speaking children ("What's that?"). LWL's two-word combinations revealed the following semantic relations: negation-action [4], assertion-object [5] and action-patient [7]. Note that in these one- to two-word (and longer sentences), LWL used nonspecific words with a Demonstrative and a Classifier (e.g., *呢個 nei1 go3* [7], *呢件 nei1 gin6* [12]) or a Demonstrative *呢 nei1* [this] and a Localizer (e.g., *呢度 nei1dou6* [here] [11]).

LWL was certainly capable of longer sentences as well. His longest sentence [9] was a benefactive Serial Verb Construction involving the verbs *幫 bong1* [help] and

着 zoek3 [wear], and it was introduced by the focus marker *係 hai6* [be]. The object of the verb *着 zoek3* [wear], however, was left unexpressed.

In the *who* question [10], the head noun for the Adjectival Modifier – that is, the sticker – was dropped. However, it could be retrieved from the discourse context. [11], a second-person imperative, included a Prepositional Phrase *喺 hai2* [at] that served as a Complement of Location to the verb *黏 nim4* [stick], whose object was unexpressed. [12] was a Subject-Adjective sentence with the adjective used in a comparative form. In addition to the generic Classifier *個 go3*, LWL used a specific Classifier *件 gin6* appropriately as well.

#2 FYS20527 (MLU100 = 2.17; GACS Grand Total = 27)

[13]* [2] *你屋企瞓覺嗰陣，你有冇呢啲㗎？*
nei5 uk1kei2 fan3gaau3 go2zan6, nei5 jau5mou5 nei1 di1 gaa3
you home sleep that-time, you have-not-have this CL SFP
(When you sleep at home, do you have this?)

[14]* *係頭先你俾你食呀？*
hai6 tau4sin1 nei5 bei2 nei5 sik6 aa4
be just-now you give you eat SFP
(Is (it) just now that you gave me (this) to eat?)

[15] *呀係咪仲有呢啲？*
aa3 hai6mai6 zung6 jau5 nei1 di1
EXC be-not-be still have this CL
((We) still have this, right?)

FYS's longest sentence was the Existential Question *有冇 jau5mou5* 'have-not-have' [13], which included a subordinate clause that ended with the Temporal Conjunction *嗰陣 go2zan6* [that time]. In this complex sentence, the use of the Possessive Construction *你屋企 nei5 uk1kei2* [your home], however, was not appropriate. In that particular context, what was needed was the *喺 hai2* [at] Preposition Phrase, *你喺屋企 nei5 hai2 uk1kei2* 'you at home' [you be at home] to specify the location encoded by the following verb *瞓覺 fan3gaau3* [sleep]. [16] revealed an adult version of the temporal subordinate clause.

[16] *你喺屋企瞓覺嗰陣 . . .*
nei5 hai2 uk1kei2 fan3gaau3 go2zan6 . . .
you at home sleep that-time
(When you sleep at home . . .)

Similar to [9] produced by #1 LWL, [14] began with the focus marker *係 hai6* [be]. There was a pronoun reversal error in the second *你 nei5* [you] in [14]. Judging from the context, it should be *你俾我食 nei5 bei2 ngo5 sik6* 'you give me eat' [you gave me (this) to eat] instead, where *俾 bei2* [give] was used as a ditransitive verb with *我ngo5* [I] as the indirect object and the direct object omitted. Despite the pronoun reversal, the rest of [14] was well formed. In fact, [14] included an Extended Ditransitive Construction (Chan, 2003), in which 俾 *bei2* [give] was followed by another verb 食 *sik6* [eat]. In the Copula question [15], FYS used the adverb 仲 *zung6* [still] to emphasize the presence of the milk they were referring to.

#3 LCK21119 (MLU100 = 2.61; GACS Grand Total = 20)

[17] *嗰個係愛嚟打波㗎。*
go2 go3 hai6 oi3lei4 daa2 bo1 gaa3
that CL be love-come hit ball SFP
(That one is used for playing ball.)

[18] *呢個愛嚟做咩㗎？*
ni1 go3 oi3lei4 zou6 me1 gaa3
this CL love-come do what SFP
(What is this used for?)

[19] *沖涼要啲呢個。*
cung1loeng4 jiu3 di1 nei1 go3
take-a-shower need some this CL
(To take a shower, (we) need some of this.)

[20] *個波喺邊呀？*
go3 bo1 hai2 bin1 aa3
CL ball at where SFP
(Where is the ball?)

[21]* *冚被嗰個呢？*
kam2 pei5 go2 go3 le1
cover duvet that CL SFP
(Where is the duvet?)
(Where is the person who covers (the baby) with the duvet?)

Incidentally, LCK21119 also used the focus marker 係 *hai6* [be] to draw attention to the clause that follows in [17]. The phrase 愛嚟 *oi3lei4* 'love-come' [used for] is often used to describe the purpose of something. It formed the key part of the prefabricated purpose question in [18]. [19] is an example of a Topic Comment sentence. The topic, encoded by the verb phase 沖涼 *cung1loeng4* 'flush-cool' (take a shower/bath), was what the following comment, needing some soap, was about. [20] illustrated a *where* question that contained only a preposition without a verb.

[21] was a rather ambiguous Particle Question and possibly an error on the part of the child. LCK and the adult were setting things up for the dolls to go to bed. The child named the pillow on request, and the adult acknowledged him and confirmed with him that the pillow was all set. It is possible that LCK intended to ask the whereabouts of the duvet that went with the pillow. A simple question like [22] would suffice. However, if LCK intended to ask for the person who covered the baby with the duvet, [21] could be seen as a Noun-Modifying

Clause (Matthews & Yip, 2017), in which the grammatical or semantic relationship between the modifying clause and the unexpressed head noun was not clearly indicated.

[22] *張被呢？*
zoeng1 pei5 le1
CL duvet SFP
(Where is the duvet?)

#4 CPY30516 (MLU100 = 3.14; GACS Grand Total = 56)

[23] *我細個嗰陣呢，*
ngo5 sai3go3 go2zan6 le1,
I small that-time PRT,
媽咪都會哩整呢啲奶奶俾我飲㗎 。
maa1mi4 dou1 wui5 le1 zing2 nei1 di1 naai1-naai1 bei2 ngo5 jam2 gaa3
mommy also would INT make this CL milk(-milk) for I drink SFP
(When I was small, my mommy would also make this kind of milk for me to drink.)

[24] *我食完飯都食埋啲皮佢㗎。*
ngo5 sik6 jyun4 faan6 dou1 sik6 maai4 di1 pei4 keoi5 gaa3
I eat finish rice also eat also CL skin it SFP
(After I finish eating, I will also eat all the apple skin.)

[25] *係呀我夜晚自己瞓㗎，食完飯。*
hai6 aa3 ngo5 je6maan5 zi6gei2 fan3 gaa3, sik6 jyun4 faan6
be SFP I night self sleep SFP, eat finish rice
(Yes, I go to sleep by myself at night, after dinner.)

[26] *我沖完涼呢都會用㗎。*
ngo5 cung1-jyun4-loeng4 le1 dou1 wui5 jung6 gaa3
I take-a-shower+finish PRT also will use SFP
(After I finish taking a shower, (I) will also use (baby powder).)

[27] *我細個，都鍾意食好多餅餅㗎。*
ngo5 sai3go3, dou1 zung1ji3 sik6 hou2 do1 beng2-beng2 gaa3
I small, also like-to eat very many biscuit(-biscuit) SFP
(When I was small, (I) also liked to eat a lot of biscuits.)

All five of CPY's sentences here involved some sort of temporal clauses. They were, however, constructed in different ways. In [23], the Temporal Conjunction 嗰陣 *go2zan6* [that time] in the subordinate clause situated the time of the event that was depicted by the following main clause. In the complex sentence [27], the Temporal Conjunction, plausibly the same 嗰陣 *go2zan6* [that time], however, was left unexpressed. In the other three sentences [24], [25] and [26], the temporal sequence of the two events was marked by the Verbal Particle 完 *jyun4* [finish]. The preference for the Verbal Particle instead of the Temporal Conjunction 之後 *zi1hau6* [after] is seen in adults as well (Matthews & Yip, 2011).

There were other features in [25] and [27] that are worth mentioning. [25] illustrated right dislocation. Typically, it is the subject or object of a clause that is moved to the end of a sentence, after the Sentence Final Particle (Matthews & Yip, 2011). In [25], the whole clause was dislocated to the right. On a different note, [27] illustrated an instance of Noun Phrase Expansion. The noun 餅 *beng2* [biscuit] was modified by the adjective 多 *do1* [many], which was further modified by the Degree Adverb 好 *hou2* [very].

Let's also examine [23] and [26] in more detail. [23] was a complex sentence not only because of the presence of a subordinate temporal clause but also because of the presence of a main clause that included the 俾 *bei2* [for] Prepositional Phrase. This phrase followed the verb 整 *zing2* [make] and preceded the verb 飲 *jam2* [drink], and both verbs involved different agents. In addition, CPY modified his verb phrase with the Modal Auxiliary 會 *wui5* [would]. He also used the Scope Adverb 都 *dou1* [also] appropriately. Regarding [26], the sentence object baby powder, which could be recovered from the discourse context, was dropped. Interjections (INT) (e.g., 哩 *le1*) were present in some of CPY's longest sentences (e.g., [23]).

#5 LHC40527 (MLU100 = 3.47; GACS Grand Total = 67)

[28] *你郁嘅定係佢自己褪後㗎，哎喲。*
nei5 juk1 ge2 ding6hai6 keoi5 zi6gei2 tan3 hau6 gaa3, ai1jo3
you move PRT or s/he self move-a-little back SFP, EXC
(Did you move, or did s/he move back him/herself?)

[29] 啊有人除咗衫好核突。
aa1 jau5 jan4 ceoi4 zo2 saam1 hou2 wat6dat6
INT have person remove ASP shirt very gross
(Argh, someone has taken his/her clothes off, and (it's) so gross.)

[30] 擳牙膏同佢沖涼先。
zit1 ngaa4gou1 tung4 keoi5 cung1loeng4 sin1
squeeze-out toothpaste help s/he take-a-shower SFP
((Let me) squeeze some toothpaste to help him/her bathe.)

[31]* 沖完涼就用梘液先。
cung1-jyun4-loeng4 zau6 jung6 gaan2jik6 sin1
take-a-shower+finish then use liquid-soap SFP
(After (one) finishes taking a shower, one uses liquid soap.)

[32] 睇吓搣唔搣到先。
tai2 haa5 mit1-m4-mit1 dou2 sin1
look ASP peel-not-peel PRT SFP
((Let me) see if (I) can peel (the fruit).)

[28] was a complex sentence involving two clauses conjoined by the Coordinating Conjunction, 定係 *ding6hai6* [or]. The Directional Particle 後 *hau6* [back] followed the verb 褪 *tan4* [move a little] to indicate the direction of the movement. [29] was a complex Subject-Adjective sentence, in which the subject was a complete clause in and of itself, and the predicate was an Adjectival Phrase 好核突

hou2 wat6dat6 [very gross]. [30] illustrated a first-person imperative sentence with a Complex Serial Verb Construction formed by stacking the three verbs 漸 *zit1* [squeeze-out], 同 *tung4* [help] and 沖涼 *cung1leong4* 'flush-cool' [take a shower/bath] together in a sequence. [31] was a grammatically complex sentence similar to [26] that #4 CPY produced, but its meaning was not consistent with world knowledge. In this sentence, the Conjunction 就 *zau6* [then], together with the Verbal Particle 完 *jyun4*, marked the temporal sequence. [32] was another first-person imperative sentence with the perception verb 睇 *tai2* [look] as the main verb. The perception verb took on a Clausal Complement, which had the structure of an A-not-A question with the reduplicated verb followed by the Resultative Particle 到 *dou2* [indicating ability]. Last but not least, sentences [30], [31] and [32] all ended with the Sentence Final Particle *sin1*. In [32], the Particle 先 *sin1* was used idiomatically with the Aspect Marker 吓 *haa5* (Matthews & Yip, 2011).

#6 CKK50015 (MLU100 = 4.27; GACS Grand Total = 92)

[33] *媽咪攞佢同我搭住被，*
maa1mi4 lo2 keoi5 tung4 ngo5 daap6 zyu6 pei5,
mommy take it help I place-on ASP duvet,
就瞓着，就唔同我冚被㗎喇。
zau6 fan3 zoek6, zau6 m4 tung4 ngo5 kam2 pei5 gaa3 laa3
then sleep PRT, then not help me cover duvet SFP SFP
(Mommy takes the duvet and helps cover me, then (she) falls asleep and cannot help put the duvet over me anymore.)

[34] 我想哩沖咗番梘之後呢，
ngo5 soeng2 le1 cung1 zo2 faan1gaan2 zi1hau6 le1,
I want(-to) INT wash) ASP soap after PRT,
我想沖番啲呢啲。
ngo5 soeng2 cung1 faan1 di1 nei1 di1
I want-to wash back some this CL
(After washing away the soap, I want to wash with some of these again.)

[35]* *媽咪成日溝溝啲奶粉嗰啲呀，*
maa1mi4 seng4jat6 kau1-kau1 di1 naai5fan2 go2 di1 aa3,
mommy all-the-time mix(-mix) some milk-power that CL SFP,
俾啲奶奶我飲。
bei2 di1 naai1naai1 ngo5 jam2
give CL milk(-milk) I drink
(Mommy makes powdered milk all the time and gives me milk to drink.)

In the complex sentence [33], CKK used the general-purpose Conjunction 就 *zau6* [then] to put three clauses in a temporal sequence. The first clause was about Mom using the duvet to cover CKK, and it involved a Complex Serial Verb Construction formed by the three verbs, 攞 *lo1* [take], 同 *tung6* [help] and 搭 *daap6* [place on]. The second clause included the verb 瞓 *fan3* [sleep], which was followed by the Resultative Particle 著 *zeok6*. The third clause included a Serial Verb Construction with the verb 同 *tung6* [help] and the verb phrase 冚被

kam2 pei5 'cover duvet' [cover the body with a duvet]. Both the second and third clauses shared the same subject with the first clause; hence, the subject was left unexpressed. In [33], CKK used the later-developing continuous Aspect Marker 住 *zyu6*.

[34] was a complex sentence with the Temporal Conjunction 之後 *zi1hau6* [after] connecting the two clauses. The verb in both clauses was modified by the Modal Auxiliary 想 *soeng2* [want to]. In the subordinate clause, CKK used the perfective Aspect Marker 咗 *zo2* to emphasize the temporal perspective established for the sentence through the use of the Conjunction. The appropriate use of the Directional Particle 番 *faan1* [back] suggested that CKK appreciated it as a homophone that carried a different semantic and syntactic function from the first syllable in the compound noun 番梘 *faan1gaan2* [soap]. There were two instances of use of Interjection in the formulation of this complex sentence.

[35] could be interpreted as an attempt by CKK to produce a sentence that looked like the main clause in [23] by #4 CPY. An adult version would be like [36] here. In [36], the *俾 bei2* [for] Prepositional Phrase followed the verb *溝 kau1* [mix] and preceded the verb *飲 jam2* [drink]. The two verbs involved two different agents. Back to [35]. As it is, the second part of [35] *俾啲奶奶我飲 bei2 di1 naai-1naai1 ngo5 jam2* [give me the milk to drink] was a well-formed Extended (*俾 bei2* [give]) Ditransitive Construction, which was discussed in relation to [14] produced by #2 FYS. The issue with [35] was that the two propositions were not properly packaged to form a coherent sentence.

[36] *媽咪成日溝啲奶粉俾我飲。*
maa1mi1 seng4jat6 kau1 di1 naai5fan2 bei2 ngo5 jam2
mommy often mix some milk-powder for I drink
(Mommy often makes some powdered milk for me to drink.)

#7 HKK50121 (MLU100 = 4.73; GACS Grand Total = 93)

[37] *但係家姐返緊學嗰時，*
daan6hai6 gaa1ze1 faan1-gan2-hok6 go2 si4,
but older-sister go-to-school+ASP that time,
就唔可以同我玩lu3！
zau6 m4 ho2ji5 tung4 ngo5 waan2 lu3
then not can with I play SFP
(But when my older sister goes to school, (she) cannot play with me!)

[38] *咁呢啲放前啲，因爲呢度係放學個房㗎。*
gam2 nei1 di1 fong3 cin4 di1, jan1wai6 nei1dou6 hai6 fong3hok6 go3 fong2 gaa3
INT this CL put front a-bit, because here be release-school CL room SFP
(These are placed a bit more to the front, because this is the room for school dismissal.)

[39] *係呀，都係咁樣，不過啲頭髮放晒落嚟㗎。*
hai6 aa3, dou1 hai6 gam2joeng2, bat1gwo3 di1 tau4faat3 fong3 saai3 lok6 lei4 gaa3
be SFP, also be like-this, but CL hair let-down all down come SFP
(Yes, (it's) also like this, but the hair is all let down.)

[40] *咁返學嗰時，*
gam2 faan1hok6 go2 si4,
INT go-to-school that time,
媽咪有時會湊我返學㗎!
maa1mi4 jau5si4 wui5 cau3 ngo5 faan1hok6 gaa3
mommy sometimes will accompany I go-to-school SFP
(When schools are in session, Mommy sometimes will take me to school!)

[41] *咁放學嗰時，*
gam2 fong3hok6 go2 si4,
INT release-school that time,
日日都係姐姐湊我，或者媽咪。
jat6jat6 dou1 hai6 ze4ze1 cau3 ngo5, waak6ze2 maa1mi4
every-day also be older-sister bring I, or mommy
(When school is dismissed, (it's) my helper who picks me up every day, or Mommy.)

In addition to temporal relations (e.g., [40] and [41]) that were observed in younger children and children with lower MLU100, HKK indicated other kinds of logical relations in his complex sentences, including concession in [37] and [39] and reason in [38]. In fact, HKK put his concessive clause in a temporal frame in [37] using the Conjunction *嗰時 go2 si4* [that time]. In the context of [37], *同 tung4* [with] was a preposition, which was then modified by the Negation Adverb *唔m4* [not] and the Modal Auxiliary *可以 ho2ji5* [can].

In the main clause of [38] and in [39], the same verb *放 fong3*, which can mean [put/place], [let go/release] or [let down] depending on the context, was used in a clause in which the object was topicalized. As Matthews and Yip (2011) pointed out, such topicalization often serves the function of Passives in English, where the object is made the subject (and thereby topic) of the clause or sentence. In the predicate of the main clause of [38], *放前啲 fong3 cin4 di1* 'put front a-bit' [place a bit more to the front], the *前 cin4* was a localizer that served as the Complement of Location for the verb. The subordinate clause of reason in [38] included a gapless Noun-Modifying Clausal Construction (Matthews & Yip, 2017) *放學個房 fong-3hok6 go3 fong2* 'release-school CL room' [the room for school dismissal]. The verb phrase *放學 fong3hok6* 'release-school' [school dismiss] related to the head noun *個房 go3 fong2* 'CL room' in an "aboutness" or semantic pragmatic sense. In [39], HKK used a Quantifying Particle *晒 saai3* [all] and two Directional Particles *落嚟 lok6 lei4* 'down come' in a row to modify the verb *放 fong3* [let down].

In [40] and [41], HKK used the frequency adverbs *有時 jau5si4* [sometimes] and *日日 jat6jat6* [every day]. In [41], HKK split the coordinated subject-noun phrase into two pieces and moved one to the end of the sentence as an afterthought.

#8 LJK50005 (MLU100 = 5.13; GACS Grand Total = 90)

[42]* 沖涼首先要哩，就係洗一陣間，
cung1loeng4 sau2sin1 jiu3 le1, zau6 hai6 sai2 jat1zan6gaan1,
take-a-shower first-of-all need(-to) INT, then be wash a-while,

然後得喇，然後哩番梘哩。
jin4hau6 dak1 laa3, jin4hau6 le1 faan1gaan2 le1
then can SFP, then INT soap INT
(To take a shower, first of all, (we) need to wash for a while, and then (it's) done, and then here's the soap.)

[43] *然後搞掂，冚番個蓋先得，*
jin4hau6 gaau2-dim6, kam2 faan1 go3 goi3 sin1 dak1,
then all-done, cover back CL lid only-then can,
唔好俾烏蠅食到。
m4hou2 bei2 wu1jing1 sik6 dou2
do-not allow/let fly eat PRT
(And then (it's) all done. (We) need to put back the lid, then (it's) okay. Don't let the flies eat (them).)

[44]* *係呀，瞓覺，唔想俾人睇，就係咁呀。*
hai6 aa3, fan3gaau3, m4 soeng2 bei2 jan4 tai2, zau6 hai6 gam2 aa3
be SFP, sleep, not want-to let/allow person see, then be like-this SFP
(Yes, when (I) sleep, (I) don't let people see (me), then (I) will be like this.)

[42] was an incomplete and non-adult sentence. It began with a Topic Comment clause that was similar to [19] produced by #3 LCK. The clause was interrupted by a self-correction, in which LJK replaced *要呢 jiu3 ne1* 'need(-to) INT' with *就係 zau6 hai6* 'just be.' The last two clauses were semantically empty with the use of only *得喇 dak1 laa3* 'can SFP' and syntactically incomplete with the bare noun *番梘 faan1gaan2* [soap] in the absence of the predicate.

[43] included a first-person imperative involving the verb *冚 kam2* [cover] and a first-person plural negative imperative in the form of *唔好 m4hou2* 'not good' [do not]. The Directional Particle *番 faan1* [back] modified the verb 冚 kam2 [cover] in the second clause; the Resultative Particle *到 dou2* [indicating ability] modified the verb *食 sik6* [eat] in the third clause. The third clause was a Pivotal Construction, with *烏蠅 wu1jing1* [fly] serving as the object of the permissive verb *俾bei2* [let/allow] and the subject of the verb *食 sik6* [eat].

In [44], there were three clauses. The first one involved the verb *瞓覺 fan3gaau3* [sleep], which marked the beginning of a sentence that expressed a temporal relationship, but the conjunction *嗰時 go2 si4* [that time] was left unexpressed. Like the third clause in [43], the third clause in [44] was a Pivotal Construction with *人 jan4* [person] serving as the object of the permissive verb *俾bei2* [let/allow] and the subject of the verb *睇 tai2* [see]. The Modal Auxiliary *想 seong2* [want to] was used to modify the verb *俾 bei2* [let/allow]. The Resultative Particle *到 dou2* was missing after the verb *睇 tai2* [see].

#9 ST40701 (MLU100 = 6.4; GACS Grand Total = 98)

[45] *你知唔知呀，我個爸爸呢傻咗，*
nei5 zi1-m4-zi1 aa3, ngo5 go3 baa4baa1 le1 so4 zo2,
you know-not-know SFP, I CL daddy PRT crazy ASP,

佢<話呢條> [//] 話我係BB嚟㗎！
keoi5 <waa6 nei1 tiu4> [//] waa6 ngo5 hai6 bi4bi1 lei4 gaa3
s/he <say this CL> [//] say I be baby SFP SFP
(Do you know, my daddy acted silly; he said I was a baby!)

[46] 拎得出嚟，嗰個就係真，
ling1 dak1 ceot1 lei4 go2 go3 zau6 hai6 zan1,
take can out come that CL then be real,
如果拎唔出嚟，嗰個就係假。
jyu4gwo2 ling1 m4 ceot1 lei4 go2 go3 zau6 hai6 gaa2
if take not out come that CL then be fake
(If (we) can take (it) out, then it is real; if (we) cannot take (it) out, then it is fake.)

[47] 如果喊嗰時呢，開咗個杯佢，
jyu4gwo2 haam3 go2 si4 le1, hoi1 zo2 go3 bui1 keoi5,
if cry that time PRT, open ASP CL cup it,
然後<俾> [//] 餵佢飲飲呀。
jin4hau6 <bei2> [//] wai3 keoi5 jam2-jam2 aa3
then <give> [//] feed s/he drink(-drink) SFP
(If and when (the baby) cries, open the cup, and then feed him the drink.)

With reference to the data for group 4 in Table 3.1, ST had a MLU100 value that was 3 standard deviations above the mean for his age. [45] began with a rhetorical Question. The second clause, which was the main clause, included a Subject-Adjective structure. The subject was in the form of a Possessive Construction *我個爸爸 ngo5 go3 baa4baa1* 'my CL daddy' [my father]. The third and subordinate clause, which gave the reason for his proposition in the previous clause, was not marked explicitly by the Conjunction 因爲 *jan1wai6* [because]. This clause also included indirect speech signaled by the verb 話 *waa6* [say].

[46] could be counted as two sentences as each could be considered an independent grammatical unit. They were, however, transcribed as one utterance in the sample for the calculation of MLU100. The reason for the decision could be that the two sentences shared a parallel structure and seemed to convey a complete thought. The sentences both conveyed a conditional relationship, which was explicitly marked by the Conjunction *就 zau6* [then] in the first sentence and the Conjunction pair *如果 jyu4gwo2* [if] and *就 zau6* [then] in the second sentence. In each sentence, the subject of the subordinate clause was not specified, and it could be inferred that it was the ST and/or the adult he was playing with. The subject of the main clause was a noun phrase without the head noun *嗰個 go2* go3 [that CL], which was likely to be a piece of toy they were playing with. In the first sentence, the verb *拎 ling1* [take] was modified by the potential particle 得 *dak1* [can], and in the second sentence, the same verb was modified by the negative counterpart of the potential particle *唔 m4* [not]. In both sentences, the verb was further modified by the two directional particles *出嚟 ceot1 lei4* [out come].

[47] was another conditional sentence, and the Temporal Conjunction 嗰時 *go2si4* [that time] was acceptable in context, although superfluous. In the sentence, the agent for the action 喊 *haam3* [cry] and that for 開 *hoi1* [open] should be different, and both were dropped. In the third and last clause, the agent and the patient for 餵 *wai3* [feed] were encoded by the pronoun 佢 *keoi5* [s/he], which does not have any markings for gender in Cantonese. The sentence might sound ambiguous out of context, but the missing arguments and the use of the pronoun could be interpreted from the discourse context and world knowledge. The one who cried would be the baby, and the one who fed the baby would be the adult. The third clause included a Pivotal Construction in which the second 佢 *keoi5* [s/he] was the object of the verb 餵 *wai3* [feed] and the subject of the verb 飲 *jam2* [drink].

#10 CWC50010 (MLU100 = 8.2; GACS Grand Total = 113)

[48]* 佢唔識蛙水，不過要剝咗，
keoi5 m4 sik1 waa1 seoi2, bat1gwo3 jiu3 mok1 zo2,
s/he not know-how-to paddle water, but need-to take-off ASP,
即係倒咗啲水先俾佢抹乾㗎。
zik1hai6 dou2 zo2 di1 seoi2 sin1 bei2 keoi5 maat3 gon1 gaa3
that-is pour ASP CL water only-then allow/give s/he wipe dry SFP
(*S/he doesn't know (how to) paddle water, and (we) need to take (his/her clothes) off, first pour out the water, then give him/her (a cloth) to dry himself/herself.)

[49]* *有泡泡都要𢯎痕，*
jau5 pou5-pou5 dou1 jiu3 ngaau1han4,
have foam(-foam) also need-to scratch-itchy,
如果啲污糟嘢先落到嚟㗎！
jyu4gwo2 di1 wu1zou1 je5 sin1 lok6 dou2 lei4 gaa3
if CL dirty thing only-then go-down PRT come SFP
(Even if there is foam, (I) still need to scratch myself; only then the dirty things can come off.)

[50]* *係呀，用個盆同你沖涼，然之後，*
hai6 aa3, jung6 go3 pun4 tung4 nei5 cung1loeng4 jin4zi1hau6,
be SFP, use CL basin help you take-a-shower then,
沖完涼就用你個盆埋裝嘢。
cung1-jyun4-loeng4 zau6 jung6 nei1 go3 pun4 maai4 zong1 je5
take-a-shower+finish then use this CL basin also hold thing
(Yes, (I) use the basin to help wash you, and after the shower, (I) will then use your basin to hold other things too.)

CWC had the highest MLU100 value in the HKU-70X corpus. His longest and complex utterances were, however, not exactly adultlike. In [48], CSW and the adult were talking about bathing the baby doll. The second clause was incomplete with the omission of both the subject-agent and the object-patient of the action *剝 mok1* [take off]. The argument drop did not seem to be justified. The third clause was ambiguous with the omission of the direct object of the ditransitive verb *俾 bei2* [give]. In fact, *幫 bong1* [help] was the more appropriate verb in this context. The word *先 sin1* [only then] was used as a Conjunction here to indicate that the second action*抹maat3* [wipe] was conditional on the first action *倒 dou2* [pour]. The verbs in this clause were modified either by the Aspect Marker *咗 zo2* or the Resultative Particle *乾 gon1* [dry]. [48] indicated an attempt to chain several related ideas into a complex sentence.

CWC seemed to struggle with the proper use of the Conditional Conjunction in [49] as it did not make sense in context. The first clause of the sentence should bring out the concession relation with the Conjunction *雖然 seoi1jin4* [although], but it was left unexpressed. In addition, in the same clause, the subject-agent for the verb *㨉痕 ngaau1han4* 'scratch-itchy' [scratch the body] was dropped. An alternative expression can be something like [51]. In [51], when the Conditional Conjunction *如果 jyu4gwo2* [if] is dropped, the last clause can be interpreted as the consequence of the action depicted in the first subordinate clause, and the sentence will be adultlike and make good sense.

[51] *雖然有泡泡，我都要㨉痕，*
seoi1jin4 jau5 pou5-pou5, ngo5 dou1 jiu3 ngaau1han4,
although have foam(-foam), I also need-to scratch-itchy,
啲污糟嘢先落到嚟㗎。
di1 wu1zou1 je5 sin1 lok6 dou2 lei4 gaa3
CL dirty thing only-then go-down PRT come SFP
(Even when there is foam, I still need to scratch myself; only then will the dirty things come off.)

[50] was a complex sentence formed by the Temporal Conjunction *然之後 jin4zi1hau6* [then]. The first clause included a Complex Serial Verb Construction formed by the verbs *用 jung6* [use], *同 tung4* [help] and *沖涼 cung1loeng4* 'flush cool' [take a shower/bath]. The use of the Quantifying Particle *埋 maai4* [also] was superfluous. Table 3.11 summarizes the forms and structures observed in the ten children.

3.8 Qualitative overviews of grammatical development: summary and future directions

In Section 3.6, we reported on the development of grammar by age group and the age of emergence and productive use of different grammatical forms and structures included in the GACS framework. In Section 3.7, we reported on grammatical forms and structures that were observed in the three to five longest non-imitative sentences in ten children with different MLU100s and GACS Grand Total scores. Items that first appeared in these ten children are marked in bold in Table 3.11, and many of these items were reported to be emerging between 2;6 and 5;11 as seen in Table 3.8. This suggests that the individual child-based analysis closely matched the findings from the analysis by age group. Three items did not appear in Table 3.11. It was not unexpected that the very short Subject-Verb and Subject-Verb-Object sentences and Particle Questions did not appear in this individual child-based analysis since only the longest sentences from the children with the lowest MLU100 of 1.49 were included in the analysis. The absence of Manner Adverbs, however, was an anomaly to be further investigated in the future.

Again, an examination of Table 3.8 and Table 3.11 in parallel shows that individual children were capable of many grammatical forms and structures that did not emerge according to group data (e.g., Relative Clause, Potential Particle, Localizer or Prepositional Phrase as a Locative Complement, Comparison of Adjectives, Sentence with a Preposition Phrase, Topic Structure, Passive Structure, a variety of questions, Coordinating, Causal and Concession Conjunction). This again suggests individual variability in language development in Cantonese-speaking children, a phenomenon that has consistently been reported in children learning English as well.

The qualitative review of individual children also revealed items that were not included in the GACS framework. These items include Sentences with Focus Verb, *what-for* questions, Clause as Sentence Subject, SVO as Sentence Subject, (Extended) Ditransitive 俾 *bei2* [give] construction, Gapless Noun Modifying Clausal Construction, First- and Second-Person Imperatives, Topic Comment Sentence, and Indirect Speech. The absence of these items in the framework can underestimate a child's grammatical capacity, especially if the focus of the analysis is only on the GACS scores. Future revision of the GACS may consider adding some of these items while striking a balance between comprehensiveness and parsimony.

Last but not least, the development of grammar as described here made use of language sample corpora collected in Hong Kong. There are two implications for this fact. First, because of Hong Kong's unique language context as discussed in Section 3.1, the developmental summaries reported here will need to be confirmed in other Cantonese-speaking communities in China, like Guangzhou and Macau. Second, while the developmental summaries might not be applicable to Cantonese-speaking bilingual children in Hong Kong and Chinese communities overseas, the quantitative and qualitative method of language sample analysis illustrated here can be adopted for these bilingual children. A case in point is MLU. Evidence reported in Yip and Matthews (2006) has subsequently shown that MLU is also a valid measure of language dominance in Cantonese-English bilingual children.

Notes

1 The term *developmental language disorder* (DLD) as defined in Bishop et al. (2017) is used in this book, despite the fact that many of the previous works discussed here used the term *specific language impairment* (SLI). Key distinctions in the definitions of DLD and SLI are reported in Chapter 4.

2 * indicates unacceptable sentences with reference to the adult standard of use. On the translation line, we provide an adult version of the sentence in English based on an interpretation of the child's intended meaning from the context.

4

GRAMMATICAL PROBLEMS IN CANTONESE-SPEAKING CHILDREN WITH DEVELOPMENTAL LANGUAGE DISORDER (DLD)

4.1 Developmental language disorder

Developmental language disorder (DLD) refers to significant difficulties in understanding, speaking and learning language. Individuals with DLD do not have a biomedical condition (e.g., hearing loss, autism spectrum disorder or intellectual disability) of which their language difficulties are a part. Individuals with DLD do sometimes have other co-occurring neurodevelopmental conditions (e.g., attention-deficit hyperactivity disorder or developmental dyslexia) that are not associated with their language difficulties.

DLD has gone by many names, including language impairment, language disorder, language delay, receptive and/or expressive language disorder or impairment, receptive and/or expressive language delay and specific language impairment (SLI). The use of multiple terms for the condition was a barrier in professional communication and public education (Bishop, 2014). SLI was the predominant term until the publication of a Delphi consensus study (Bishop et al., 2017), after which the term DLD was recommended. One key distinction between SLI and DLD is the cut-off score for the nonverbal IQ criteria. SLI requires a score of 85 or above (Leonard, 2014) and DLD a score of at least 70 (Bishop et al., 2017). A child with significant language difficulties is considered to have DLD if s/he does not have an IQ score that normally qualifies a person as having an intellectual disability: that is, 70 or below. An additional criterion for DLD is that the language difficulties should have a functional impact on the child's everyday life. Throughout this book, the term DLD, instead of the original term SLI as used in some of the cited works, is adopted.

The same diverse set of English terms and their translations and acronyms are used in research and clinical practice in Chinese contexts. In 2021, the Hong Kong Speech Therapists Association adopted a document (Wong et al., 2021)

DOI: 10.4324/9780367824013-4

prepared by the special interest group on terminology for child language disorders. The document summarizes diagnostic distinctions between DLD and language disorders associated with a biomedical condition as discussed in Bishop et al. (2017). The document also includes the Chinese terms for the different diagnostic labels.

4.2 DLD in Cantonese

In English-speaking countries, the prevalence of DLD is reported to be 11.1% (Tomblin et al., 1997) and 7.6% (Norbury et al., 2016). Despite the lack of prevalence data in Hong Kong, children with DLD are diagnosed and treated by professionally trained speech-language therapists. Diagnosis is made objectively using evidence collected from several sources, including the two omnibus standardized norm-referenced language tests developed specifically for Cantonese-speaking children in Hong Kong. These relatively recent tests include reports of adequate reliability, validity and diagnostic accuracy. The TOPOL is appropriate for use with preschoolers between 2;6 and 5;11 (Child Assessment Service, 2019), and the HKCOLAS is designed for school-aged children between 5;00 to 10;11 (T'sou et al., 2006).

4.3 Linguistic characteristics of DLD in Cantonese: an overview

Research on Cantonese-speaking children with DLD did not begin until the mid-1990s. The small body of studies involved primarily preschool children, with the exception of To et al. (2010). As a Sino-Tibetan language, Cantonese is typologically very different from Indo-European languages like English. One can easily draw this conclusion from Chapter 1. Linguistic characteristics that distinguish children with DLD from typically developing children, therefore, are not the same for Cantonese and English. In this section, we will provide an overview of the linguistic characteristics of Cantonese DLD and report on cross-linguistic comparisons with English DLD where appropriate.

A brief discussion on the research methodology typically used in studies of linguistic characteristics of DLD is needed here. In addition to a group of typically developing age peers (AM), a typically developing group of younger children who are sometimes also matched with children in the DLD group on a language measure (Y-(LM)) is also included. The inclusion of an AM group allows researchers to ascertain that the language form or structure under investigation is a problem only for children with DLD and not their age peers. On the other hand, the Y-(LM) group helps researchers rule out the chosen matching variable as an explanation for any observed differences between the DLD and the Y-(LM) groups. The most common control variables are mean length of utterance and the raw score on an omnibus language test. Let's say the DLD group scores lower than the younger control group who are matched on a test's raw scores on the use of the past tense

-ed morpheme. It means that the DLD group's worse performance is not a result of a general depression in language knowledge and use. The past tense *-ed* morpheme is therefore identified as a form of exceptional difficulty for children with DLD, and an explanation for this exceptional difficulty is called for. While children with DLD will differ from children in the AM group on most language forms and structures, they do not necessarily do worse than children in the Y-(LM) group on all these forms and structures.

4.3.1 Vocabulary, lexical diversity and mean length of utterance

Cantonese-speaking preschool children with DLD used fewer types of words (Klee et al., 2004; Stokes & Fletcher, 2000; Wong et al., 2010) and produced shorter utterances in conversation on average (Klee et al., 2004; Wong et al., 2004) than their AM peers, in much in the same way as children learning English (Rice et al., 2010). To et al. (2010) reported that the DLD group, which included children from a wide age range from 5;3 to 12;5, used fewer of the target sophisticated words in a story retell task than their AM peers. This set of studies confirms that DLD does share some universal, albeit general, features across languages.

4.3.2 Syntactic complexity and referencing in narrative discourse

The goal of To et al.'s (2010) study was to document the diagnostic accuracy of the narrative retell subtest of the HKCOLAS. Analyses of the results revealed that school-aged children with DLD scored lower than their AM peers on a measure of syntactic complexity in the story retell task. In fact, this measure was the best among the four candidate measures that differentiated children with and without DLD. The measure of syntactic complexity included relative clause, preverbal manner modifier, clausal complement and prepositional phrase. As it was not the goal of the study, it remained unclear which of these structures were more difficult for children with DLD.

Another measure in the HKCOLAS narrative retell task that was reported to distinguish school-aged children with DLD and their AM peers was character referencing (To et al., 2010). Children with DLD were not able to use explicit nominal forms when switching and introducing referents in their stories as well as their AM peers.

4.3.3 Conjunctions

A third measure in the narrative retell task that showed a statistically significant difference between the DLD and the AM groups was the use of Conjunctions (To et al., 2010). School-aged children with DLD used fewer conjunctions in their sentences than their AM peers, although this group difference was of least practical significance, given its small effect size.

4.3.4 Aspect Markers

A number of studies on Cantonese DLD examined linguistic forms and structures that allowed testing of competing theoretical explanations of DLD. These forms and structures were Aspect Markers, Passives and Questions. Aspect Markers were the most studied linguistic form in Cantonese DLD (Fletcher et al., 2005; Stokes & Fletcher, 2000, 2003). Fletcher et al. (2005) give three reasons for it. One is that grammatical markers with temporal meanings were the focus of much research on DLD. In fact, evidence suggested that persistent difficulties in tense morphemes and person-agreement morphemes were clinical markers of DLD in English-speaking children (Rice et al., 1999). Two is that because the *-ing* progressive Aspect Marker appeared rather early in English-speaking children with DLD, there was little research attention on the investigation of aspect (but see Leonard et al., 2003). Last but not least, in English and in many languages investigated, aspectual marking does not occur independently of tense on the verb form. Cantonese, however, marks only aspect but not tense on its verbs and adjectives, thus providing a useful context to examine children with DLD's potential problems in aspectual marking in isolation.

Data from a variety of tasks, including conversation with an adult (Stokes & Fletcher, 2000; Stokes & Fletcher, 2003), sentence repetition and video narration (Stokes & Fletcher, 2003) and an experimental task (Fletcher et al., 2005) confirmed that Cantonese-speaking children with DLD did worse than their AM peers. In fact, Cantonese-speaking children with DLD had more difficulties with the perfective and continuous Aspect Markers under study in Fletcher et al. (2005) than children in the Y-(LM) group as well.

Cantonese being a language that is morphologically extremely sparse, its Aspect Markers do not contrast person or number within a paradigm and, hence, do not provide valid cues for the identification or marking of grammatical relations in a sentence. In addition, aspectual marking is grammatically optional and pragmatically determined in Cantonese. Verbs can appear without an Aspect Marker, and the sentence can still be grammatical. The use of Aspect Markers is determined by the speaker's choice on whether to restrict the listener's interpretation of the event, the speaker's viewpoint of the internal temporal structure of the event encoded by the verb and the speaker's knowledge of the inherent semantics of the verb (i.e., situation aspect) with which the Aspect Marker collocates. For Cantonese-speaking children with DLD, their problems with the grammatically optional Aspect Markers can, therefore, have a pragmatic and/or semantic origin, as suggested in the findings reported in Stokes and Fletcher (2000, 2003). In both studies, children restricted the target Aspect Marker(s) with a small set of verbs denoting the temporal properties of events or states of that were consistent with the semantics of the Aspect Marker(s).

4.3.5 Passives

Leonard et al. (2006) examined for the first time the production of Passives in Cantonese-speaking children with DLD. Again, in keeping with being a morphologically sparse language, the verb in Cantonese Passives is not morphologically marked for tense or agreement. Unlike English, there is no distinction between the verb forms in Cantonese Active and Passive sentences. Cantonese-speaking children did worse than their AM peers, but the difference did not reach statistical significance. More importantly, they performed at a comparable level to their Y-(LM) controls. In the same report, results from English-speaking children with DLD were also presented. English-speaking children with DLD, however, did worse than both their AM and Y-(LM) controls.

4.3.6 Questions

In English, the *wh* word in Questions can only occur in the initial position. In a well-formed *wh*-object question, the *wh*-word moves from its interpreted position (i.e., the object noun phrase) to the initial position of the Question. Such a movement, however, is not required in *wh*-subject questions. English-speaking children with DLD were shown to have more problems with *wh*-object questions than *wh*-subject questions when compared to children in the Y-(LM) group (van der Lely & Battell, 2003) as they treated movement as being optional. In Cantonese, *wh* words in both subject and object Questions remain in situ, occupying the same position as in declarative sentences. Some linguists argue that movement of constituents is not involved in Cantonese *wh* questions. It therefore could be predicted that *wh* questions should not be a problem for Cantonese-speaking children with DLD. But this was not what was found. Cantonese-speaking children with DLD showed the same pattern of results with poorer performance in *who*-object than *who*-subject questions (Wong et al., 2004) as their English-speaking counterparts. Alternative proposals calling attention to the role of animacy of the referents of the *wh* word and input frequency were offered for future investigation of *wh* questions in Cantonese-speaking children with DLD.

4.3.7 Modal Auxiliaries

In Leonard et al. (2007), the of use of Modal Auxiliaries in Cantonese-speaking children with DLD and their English-speaking counterparts was examined in three studies. This was the first study on the use of Modal Auxiliaries to express different semantic notions in Cantonese-speaking children with DLD. There were some earlier works on Modal Auxiliaries in English-speaking children with DLD, but it remained unclear whether their performance in Modal Auxiliaries could have been confounded by their persistent problems with tense.

In the study that examined the same Modal Auxiliary for ability in both the past (i.e., "could") and non-past (i.e., "can") contexts, English-speaking children with DLD were found to do significantly worse in the use of the past "could" than the non-past "can," a result not found in the two typically developing control groups. The interaction effect also revealed another important finding. Children with DLD did worse than children in the Y-(LM) group in the past "could" but not the non-past "can." This pattern of results suggested that Modal Auxiliaries, at least the one for communicating the semantic notion of ability, did not seem to be an area of exceptional difficulty for English-speaking children with DLD per se and that their problems with tense extended to Modal Auxiliaries.

The study on Cantonese-speaking children with DLD provided supportive evidence to the prediction that if Modal Auxiliaries did not carry tense, as in Cantonese, they were not going to be difficult for children with DLD. Cantonese-speaking children with DLD showed no difference in the use of the ability 識 *sik1* [know how to] and permissive 可以 *ho2ji3* [can/could, may/might] Modal Auxiliaries compared to the AM and Y-(LM) controls in experimental tasks presented in the past and non-past contexts.

4.3.8 Noun Classifiers

The first attempt to investigate language-specific features of DLD in Cantonese-speaking speaking children was a study on noun Classifiers (Stokes & So, 1997). Noun Classifiers do not exist in English per se, and the nearest English form is words used in counting or numerating (e.g., "pairs," as in "two pairs of gloves"). There are over 60 Classifiers in Cantonese (Matthews & Yip, 2011), and in many contexts, a Classifier is grammatically obligatory in a noun phrase. One such context is the presence of a quantifier or numeral before the head noun, as in [1] and [2]. Classifiers are chosen on the basis of the "distinctive features of shape, natural kind and function" (p. 109) of the object noun they modify. The most common and generic Classifier is 個 *go3*, which can be used with all kinds of words referring to people and with individual items in place of a more specific Classifier.

[1] 每個人
mui5 go3 jan4
every CL person
(every person)

[2] 三條裙
saam1 tiu4 kwan4
three CL dress
(three dresses)

In Stokes and So (1997), children were asked to label objects presented in sets. The sets of objects created a context that required the use of a numeral, which in turn obligated a Classifier to precede the head noun. There was a marked variability in the total percentage correct and the percentage correct of each of the nine Classifiers in the 37-item task in the group of children with DLD and their AM controls. Group effects were not statistically significant, but there were qualitative differences in the two groups' error responses. The predominant pattern in the AM controls was substitution, and the most frequently observed substitute was the generic Classifier 個 *go3*. Omission of Classifiers was rather rare. Children with DLD, however, showed a more diverse set of errors. While substitution was also the predominant pattern children with DLD, omission errors were 27 times higher than the level observed in children in the AM group.

4.3.9 Summary

Table 4.1 summarizes findings from published studies investigating Cantonese-speaking children's use of specific language forms and structures relative to the AM and younger Y-(LM) controls. Among all the specific language forms and structures studied so far, Cantonese-speaking children with DLD did worse than the AM group in Conjunctions, Aspect Markers, *Who*-Object Questions, and also noun Classifiers, albeit in qualitative terms. When compared with the Y-(LM) group, they did worse in Aspect Markers and *Who*-Object Questions. Evidence so far did not show quantitative differences between children with either control groups on Passives, *Who*-Subject Questions, and Modal Auxiliaries. But then, when referring to the GACS discussed in Chapter 2, there are many forms and structures in Cantonese that have not been examined in children with DLD across a wide age range. But where should we look, and how should we start?

TABLE 4.1 Summary of published findings on the linguistic characteristics of DLD in Cantonese

	Statistical comparison with typically developing same-age peers	*Statistical comparison with typically developing younger and/or language-matched controls*
Conjunctions	DLD worse	—
Aspect Markers (Fletcher et al., 2005)	DLD worse	DLD worse
Aspect Markers (Stokes & Fletcher, 2000)	—	DLD not different, but qualitative analysis showed restricted distribution of the Aspect Marker across verbs
Aspect Markers (Stokes & Fletcher, 2003)	DLD not different in sentence repetition; worse in video narrative and conversation. Qualitative analysis showed restricted distribution of the Aspect Marker across verbs	—
Passives	DLD not different	DLD not different
Who-Subject Questions	DLD not different	DLD not different
Who-Object Questions	DLD worse	DLD worse
Modal Auxiliaries	DLD not different	DLD not different
Classifiers	DLD differed in error patterns	—

4.4 Further investigation of the linguistic characteristics of DLD in Cantonese: a proposal

First, develop knowledge of a descriptive framework of Cantonese grammar and an understanding of how different linguistic features are used to communicate who does what to whom and how the basic meaning of a sentence can be elaborated. Second, specify the age range of children who have DLD for the investigation. This is important because DLD is a developmental problem, and its linguistic manifestations change with age. Children with DLD can show problem X at age A and problem Y at age B. The literature has reported, however, that a problem can persist for some time in children with DLD. Problems with tense and agreement marking in English-speaking children with DLD (see Leonard, 2014 for an overview) are a case in point. Third, identify what language forms and structures are observed in most typically developing children in this age range from, say, conversational and/or narrative samples. Fourth, observe if individual children with DLD demonstrate errors in these developmentally appropriate forms and structures. These errors are potential items of difficulty for children in this age range as a group. Fifth, collect data on these forms and structures from children with DLD and their AM controls using experimental tasks to ascertain that these errors are observed in a majority of children with DLD and hence, likely to be potential clinical markers. Sixth, given positive results, include an additional group of Y-(LM) control in a larger study to examine if the forms and structures are exceptional items of difficulty on which the DLD group does worse than the Y-(LM) group.

How far one goes with this proposal depends on one's goals. To identify clinical markers for use in the screening and diagnosis of DLD, one may pause at step 5. One will examine statistically the screening and diagnostic accuracy of the markers before they are used in evidence-based clinical practice. Note that not all the potential clinical markers will have high accuracy, given that children with DLD are rather heterogeneous in the language difficulties they demonstrate. In search of an explanation of DLD at the cognitive and/or the biological level, the sixth step is a methodology that has been used for some time, although arguments were raised on its drawbacks (Plante et al., 1993).

To conclude, systematic investigations of the linguistic characteristics of DLD in Cantonese are critically important for clinical assessment and intervention. These investigations also contribute to the cross-linguistic understanding of DLD, which is an impairment that affects all children regardless of the language(s) they are exposed to. This understanding will eventually lead to solving the mystery of the human capacity for language learning.

4.5 The linguistic profile of a six-year-old Cantonese-speaking child with DLD

In this section, we describe the language of CY, a 6;4 girl with DLD, in terms of form, content and use (Bloom & Lahey, 1978). In the description of form, we use the *Grammatical Analysis of Cantonese Samples* (GACS) framework as detailed in Chapter 2. We will also examine her errors in detail.

CY was diagnosed as having a "language delay" when she was 3;6 at one of the comprehensive assessment centers in Hong Kong. She received several blocks of therapy with different service providers after her diagnosis. At 6;7, CY received a re-assessment of her language skills. In the HKCOLAS, she received a standard score of −2.4 SD on Cantonese Grammar, 2.1 SD on Textual Comprehension, −0.8 SD on Word Definition, −2.0 SD on Story Retell and −2.6 SD on Expressive Nominal Vocabulary. Since she scored lower than −1.25 in more than two subtests, she failed the standardized norm-referenced test.

CY was a generally happy child who did not seem to be too aware of her problems. Her parents, however, were concerned about her language skills and decided to have her repeat the final year of preschool. In Hong Kong, most children attend half-day or full-day preschool five days a week at three years of age and start primary one at six.

There were no concerns with CY's hearing or psychosocial or cognitive development in her preschool years. A year after CY started primary school, the school educational psychologist related to the parents that she was low average in her cognitive skills and that she had developmental dyslexia. Following the CATALSE framework, CY was considered to have DLD that co-occurred with developmental dyslexia. CY's younger sister was also diagnosed as having language disorder in her preschool years.

When CY was 6;4, the speech-language therapist who had known her and her family for a few years engaged in conversation with her while playing with a toy house. The 20-minute conversation was videotaped and transcribed in Chinese characters. The transcript is attached in Appendix A. A completed score sheet of the language sample analysis using the GACS is attached in Appendix B.

4.5.1 CY's language use

Pragmatics is the use of language in conversation and social interactions. Observation of her conversational interaction with a familiar adult suggested that CY's language use was appropriate for her age. She initiated and maintained topics and was responsive to communication bids. She adopted an appropriate speech register for different toy figures during play. Her sentences performed a range of communicative functions, including regulatory as well as interactional. As is clear from the language sampled analysis, she used eight different Sentence Final Particles to indicate different speech act types and evidentiality of the sentence, as well as her attitudes, moods and emotions towards the situation.

4.5.2 CY's language content

Language content refers to knowledge and use of words and word relations. In the conversational sample, CY was not able to name a common object *梳化 so1faa2*

[sofa] or a less familiar object *火爐 fo2lou4* [fireplace]. Excerpt [3][1] illustrates how she took a few turns to describe the sofa instead of naming it. CY's attempt to refer to the fireplace will be discussed under Noun Phrase Expansion later in this chapter. CY's difficulty in vocabulary was consistent with her performance in the Expressive Nominal Vocabulary subtest in the HKCOLAS, scoring 2.6 SD below the mean for her age.

[3]

INV: *不過我哋擺好晒啲嘢先請佢出嚟啦。咦！依個係 . . .*
(But let's put everything away first and then ask him to come out. Look! This is a . . .)
INV: {pointing to the sofa}
CHI: *彈嘅。*
daan6 ge3
bounce SFP
((We) bounce on (it).)
INV: *哦，我知啦。你梗係平時喺度咁樣彈嘅。* (with laughter)
(Ah, I see. You must bounce on it here like this often.)
CHI: *坐低嘅。*
co5 dai1 ge3
sit down SFP
((We) sit on (it).)
INV: *坐低嘅，咁呢個係 . . .*
(We sit on it. And this is a . . .)
CHI: *挨住嘅。*
aai1 zyu6 ge3
lean ASP SFP
((We) lean on (it).)
INV: *係呀，挨住嘅。*
(Yes, we lean on it.)
CHI: *呢個X挨住。*
nei1 go3 X aai1 zyu6
this CL X lean ASP
(This one (we) lean on.)
INV: *呢個係梳化。*
(This one is a sofa.)
CHI: 梳化。
so1faa2
sofa
(Sofa.)

The two next excerpts illustrate CY's difficulties with word definition as well. They provide converging evidence for her low performance in the Word Definition subtest in the HKCOLAS, scoring 0.8 SD below the age mean. Excerpt [4] illustrates how CY defined beds.

[4]

INV: *係呀，床要嚟做咩㗎？*
(Yes. What is the bed for?)
CHI: *擺喺度。*
baai2 hai2 dou6
put at PRT
((We) put (it) here.)
INV: *好呀。咁要嚟做咩㗎，張床？*
(Sure. What is it for, the bed?)
CHI:*[2] *我哋呢，夜晚哩，係哩，瞓覺嘅。*
ngo5dei6 le1, je6maan5 le1, hai6 le1, fan3gaau3 ge3
we PRT, night INT, be INT, sleep SFP
(At night, . . . we . . . sleep (there).)

For objects, preschool and early primary school children usually provide information on their functions in the definition (To et al., 2013), using the simple phrase *要嚟 jiu3lei4* 'want-come' [used for] or *愛嚟 oi3lei4* 'love-come' [used for]. Instead of this phrase, CY used the inappropriate copula verb *係hai6* [be]. To define *床 cong4* [bed], a typically developing child would produce a sentence like [5], which includes the Temporal Conjunction *嗰陣時 go2zan6si4* [that time].

[5] *我哋夜晚嗰陣時要嚟瞓覺嘅。*
ngo5dei6 je6maan5 go2zan6si4 jiu3lei4 fan3gaau3 ge3
we night that-time want-come sleep SFP
((When it is nighttime, we use (it) for sleeping.)

In an attempt to define lamps, CY produced [6], which includes an unnecessary Modal Auxiliary 要 *jiu3* [need to], which was possibly a self-correction. The sentence was also interrupted with frequent Interjections, which were not uncommon in CY's sentences, as we shall see later. A grammatically appropriate sentence produced by a typically developing child would look like [7]. A closer look at CY's sentence [6], however, shows that she did not actually define lamps and give their proper function, which is giving light when it is dark. Instead, she constructed a sentence with the word "lamp."

[6]

INV: *要嚟做咩嘢呀？*
(What is (the lamp) for?)
CHI:* *我哋哩，要哩，瞓覺哩，要熄燈嘅。*
ngo5dei6 le1, jiu3 le1, fan3gaau3 le1, jiu3 sik1 dang1 ge3
we INT, need-to INT, sleep INT, need-to turn-off lamp SFP
((When) we go to sleep, we turn off the lamp.)

[7] *我哋瞓覺要熄燈嘅。*
ngo5dei2 fan3gaau3 jiu3 sik1 dang1 ge3
we sleep need-to turn-off lamp SFP
(When we go to sleep, we have to turn off the lamp.)

To conclude, it was clear from test results and the transcript of her conversation that CY had problems with language content, especially in vocabulary. She lacked the words for many objects, some common and some less familiar. CY's definition revealed that she probably had adequate knowledge of the world but not the language to directly and effectively communicate that knowledge.

4.5.3 CY's language form

Language form refers to knowledge of the rules of language, including the domains of syntax, morphology and phonology. CY demonstrated inconsistent errors with some speech sounds in some words in a formal test of articulation, the Cantonese Articulation Test (Cheung et al., 2006). CY sometimes slurred her words; hence, some of her syllables were marked as unintelligible in the transcript. Her speech was intelligible to familiar individuals about 95% of the time.

Syntax and morphology were major problems for CY. We will examine her language form following the structure of the GACS framework section by section, except that Conjunctions are discussed with Sentence Structures.

Noun Phrase Expansion

CY did not expand many of her noun phrases, which could be related to the here-and-now context in conversation. CY used two different Classifiers, one of which was the generic Classifier *個 go3*. The Classifier *張 zeong1* was omitted when CY referred to *櫈 dang3* [chair] in an error sentence [8]. This observation was consistent with results reported in Stokes and So (1997). While substitution error was seen in typically developing children, omission of Classifiers was more common in children with DLD.

[8]* *唔啱依個好大櫈嘅。*
m4 ngaam1 ji1 go3 hou2 daai6 dang3 ge3
not right this CL very big chair SFP
((It's) not right. This chair is very big.)

CY used the *喺 hai2* Prepositional Modifier to expand the noun in two instances. One of these instances is given in [9]. In [9], the head noun *櫃 gwai6* [cupboard] was first slurred and then was added back to the sentence after the first Sentence Final Particle *囉 lo1*. This could be interpreted as an instance of word retrieval problem.

[9] *喺屋企嘅XX囉櫃囉*
hai2 uk1kei2 ge3 XX lo1 gwai6 lo1
at home PRT XX SFP cupboard SFP
(the closet that is at home)

There was no proper use of Relative Clauses in CY's conversational sample. When she referred to the *火爐 fo2lo4* [fireplace], she made an attempt to produce a Relative Clause with omission of the generic head noun *嘢 je5* [thing] in [10]. The omission of the head noun was acceptable but the omission of the Preposition *喺 hai2* [at] before the Localizer 中間 *zung1gaan1* [middle] was not.

[10]* *有火中間嗰個囉XX。*
jau5 fo2 zung1gaan1 go2 go3 lo1 XX
have fire middle that CL SFP XX
(The one that has fire in the middle.)

As seen in the GACS score sheet in Appendix B, CY also used Possessive Constructions and Adjectival Modifiers appropriately once. The use of Nominal Modifiers and Locative Modifiers was not observed. Given that conversation about here-and-now objects is not usually conducive to Noun Phrase Expansion, there is a need to further examine CY's ability to modify nouns in other discourse genres. In fact, CY's narrative retell sample from the HKCOLAS would provide additional information on her use of noun phrases, as well as other aspects of language form. Interested readers may refer to the *Grammatical Analysis of Narrative Samples* (GACN) framework (Wong et al., 2022), which is an adaptation of the GACS framework for the analysis of narratives, and CY's narrative retell transcript and GACN score sheet (Wong, 2022) for details.

Verb phrase expansion

As seen in Appendix B, CY used three different Modal Auxiliaries: two are early developing *可以 ho2ji5* [can/could, may/might] and *會 wui5* [will/would]), and one is later developing (*要 jiu3* [want to, need to]). She also used three different Aspect Markers, two early developing (*咗 zo2* and *住 zyu6*) and one later developing (*吓 haa5*). So both Modal Auxiliaries and Aspect Markers were productive word classes for CY. [11] illustrates CY's correct use of *跌 dit3* [fall] with the Aspect Marker *咗 zo2*.

[11] *BB 跌咗。*
BB dit3 zo2
baby fall SPF
(The baby has fallen off (the chair).)

Despite evidence of productive use, errors were noted in the use of individual members of these word classes of Modal Auxiliaries and Aspect Markers, albeit inconsistently. [12] illustrated an instance of incorrect use of the Aspect Marker *咗 zo2*. [12a] was a grammatically appropriate sentence, but it was inconsistent with one's expectation given the discourse context. In the context of [12a], a typically developing child, however, would say *會跌 wui5 dit3* [will/would fall] instead of

跌咗 dit3 zo2 'fall ASP' [have fallen]. In fact, this was what CY said in her next speaking turn in [12b]. This provided evidence that CY meant to talk about the possibility rather than the completion of an action.

[12]

INV: *我坐 . . . 我坐呢邊。*
(I sit . . . I sit on this side.)

CHI*: *唔好呀，呢個BB㗎，跌咗㗎。* [a]
m4hou2 aa3, nei1 go3 BB gaa3, dit3 zo2 gaa3
do-not SFP, this CL baby SFP, fall ASP SFP
(Don't. This baby has fallen off (the chair).)

INV: *我坐 . . . 枱上面。*
(I sit . . . on the table.)

CHI: *唔好呀，會跌㗎。* [b]
m4hou2 aa1, wui2 dit3 gaa3
do-not SFP, will fall SFP
(Don't. (The baby) will fall off (the chair).)

On the basis of [11] and [12a], one may suggest that CY used *跌咗 dit3 zo2* 'fall ASP' [have fallen] as an unanalyzed item. In fact, Stokes and Fletcher (2000, 2003) did show that children with DLD restricted the use of some Aspect Markers with a small set of verbs.

How do we explain this pattern of inconsistent use in CY? Given instances of proper use of *跌咗 dit3 zo2* 'fall ASP' [have fallen] and *會跌 wui5 dit3* [will/would fall] in other contexts during the conversation, it is not likely that CY lacked knowledge of the forms for what she wanted to say. It is, however, possible that in situations when the demand for sentence formulation was high – for example, in the production of a longer sentence [12a] – the unanalyzed item was activated and produced before the proper phrase was constructed.

In addition to the verb *跌 dit3* [fall], CY used *咗 zo2* productively with three other verbs, *調轉 diu6zyun3* [switch], *沖 cung1* [flush] and *撞 zong6* [hit]. While CY's single instance of use of *調轉 diu6zyun3* [switch] and *沖 cung1* [flush] were both appropriate, she made a mistake with *撞咗 zong6 zo2* 'hit ASP' [have hit] twice, in much the same way as *跌咗 dit3 zo2* 'fall ASP' [have fallen] in [12]. (See [13].)

[13]

INV: *係喎，有人喺度喎。咁呀，我擺另一邊啦。*
(That's right, there is somebody here. Right, I put (it) on the other side.)

CHI:* *但係依道門呢，撞咗人呀。*
daan6hai6 ji1 dou6 mun4 le1, zong6 zo2 jan4 aa3
but this CL door PRT hit ASP person SFP
(But this door has hit someone.)

A typically developing child would use the modal auxiliary 會 *wui5* [will] + verb + the Resultative particle 到 *dou2* [indicating ability] construction, as in [14], to indicate that the therapist's suggested placement of the sofa would result in the action encoded by the verb 撞 *zong6* [hit]. There were two possible explanations for CY's error: first, an issue with the use of a semantically appropriate combination of Modal Auxiliaries and Verbal Particles and second, an issue with the subtle semantic distinction between the perfective Aspect Marker 咗 *zo2* and the Resultative Verbal Particle 到 *dou2* [indicating ability] as discussed in Chapter 1.

[14] *但係依道門會撞到人呀*
daan6hai6 ji1 dou6 mun4 wui5 zong6 dou2 jan4 aa3
but this CL door will hit PRT person SFP
(But this door will hit someone.)

CY made another substitution error just like [13] in [15]. This time, the error involved the delimitative Aspect Marker 吓 *haa5* instead of the perfective Aspect Marker 咗 *zo2*. At the time CY was producing the sentence, the therapist was suggesting that she put the television set upstairs. CY confirmed the suggestion and produced the sentence in [15]. The fact that the therapist used the Resultative Particle 到 *dou2* [indicating ability] in her sentence after CY's reveals that it was the more appropriate postverbal modifier in that context but not the Aspect Marker 吓 *haa5*.

[15]
CHI:* *望吓哩出邊嘅。*
mong6 haa5 le1 ceot1bin6 ge3
look ASP INT outside SFP
(Have a look at the outside.)
INV: 又可以望到出面睇風景。
((We) can also look outside and see the scenery.)

Aspect Markers and Verbal Particles are syntactically optional, so omission errors are less obvious. [16] illustrated an error from CY. In CY's second next turn after this error sentence, she said that the older brother was getting up. This subsequent sentence confirmed the fact that the older brother was sleeping, and the use of the continuous Aspect Marker 緊 *gan2* made the sentence semantically and pragmatically more complete.

[16]
INV: *好呀！姐姐，姐姐我哋玩咩嘢呀？*
(Good! Older sister, what do we play?)
CHI:* *哥哥呢瞓覺呀，*
go4go1 le1 fan3gaau3 aa1
older-brother PRT sleep SFP

我哋叫佢哩一齊玩吖。
ngo5dei2 giu3 keoi5 le1 jat1cai4 waan2 aa1
we ask him INT together play SFP
(The older brother is sleeping. Let's ask him to play with us.)

[17] illustrates CY's omission of the Verbal Particle *埋 maai4* [also]/[along]. The therapist's sentences before and after CY's suggest that the presence of the Verbal Particle would make the meaning of her sentence more semantically complete.

[17]

INV: 家姐，等埋我呀。
gaa1ze1, dang2 maai4 ngo5 aa3
older-sister, wait also me SFP
(Older sister, wait for me to get there too.)

CHI:* 我等你。
ngo5 dang2 nei5
I wait you
(I'll wait for you.)

INV: 家姐，等埋呀。
gaa1ze1, dang2 maai4 aa3
older-sister, wait also SFP
(Older sister, wait for me to get there too.)

Regarding modifiers that appear after the verb, CY used three different Aspect Markers, three different Resultative Particles, four different Directional particles or particle combinations and the negative Potential particle *唔 m4* [not] appropriately. CY also talked about location with the use of a complement after the verb. In her Complements of Location, CY used a Localizer (e.g., *呢度 nei1dou6* [here], *度 dou6* [PRT], *出邊 ceot1bin6* [outside]) without the noun in four out of five times. As is clear from Appendix B, Descriptive Complements and Complements of Extent were not observed. Regarding modifiers that appear before the verb, CY used three different Modal Auxiliaries, four different Manner Adverbs, two different Negation Adverbs, and one Degree Adverb.

Last but not least, in Cantonese, the same syllable can have two different, and sometimes closely related, meanings and take up more than one syntactic role without a change in form. An example is the syllable *開 hoi1*. It can be a verb that means [open]/[turn on], or it can be a Directional Particle meaning [away]. In [18], CY used *開 hoi1* [open] as a verb when it should have been a Directional Particle following the missing verb *拉laai1* [pull]. The sentence was in error as the improper use of the syllable led to difficulties for her listeners in interpreting what she meant. A typically developing child would produce a sentence like [19].

[18]* *開櫈先。*
hoi1 dang3 sin1
open chair SFP
((Let me) pull the chair away (from the table) first.)

[19] *拉開張櫈先。*
laai1 hoi1 zoeng1 dang3 sin1
pull away CL chair SFP
((Let me) pull the chair away (from the table) first.)

To conclude, CY used various forms to modify the verb(s) in her sentences, adding information on possibility, manner, negation, result, direction, extent and location of the action. Errors, however, were observed in the use of some of these forms. CY had difficulty making the subtle distinction between the perfective Aspect Marker *咗 zo2* and the Modal Auxiliary *會 wui5* [will/would] in the combined use of the Modal Auxiliary *會 wui5* [will] and the Resultative Particle *到 dou2* [indicating ability] and in making the subtle distinction between the Resultative Particle *到 dou2* [indicating ability] and Aspect Marker *咗 zo2*. On occasion, CY omitted the Aspect Marker *緊 gan2* and Verbal Particle *埋 maai4* [also]/[along]. Last but not least, CY had trouble with the proper use of words that have a dual role as verbs and Verbal Particles.

Sentence Structures

As shown in CY's GACS summary sheet in Appendix B, she appropriately used at least three different Verb-Object Structures, Subject-Verb-Object Structures, Subject-Verb Structures, Subject-Adjective Structures and Existential Constructions, suggesting good control of these basic sentence types. She produced one Comparative Construction, one Pivotal Construction, one sentence with the *同 tung4* [with]/[together with] Prepositional Phrase, one sentence with the *到 dou3* [arrive at] Prepositional Phrase, two sentences with the *喺 hai2* [at] Prepositional Phrase, three sentences with a Clausal Complement and four simple Serial Verb Constructions. This list suggests that CY had a rather diverse repertoire of syntactic constructions at her disposal in conversation. Having said that, not all CY's sentences were grammatically appropriate.

a. Omission of the verb

In [20], [21] and [22], the verb is absent. All three sentences were produced when CY and the therapist were putting different objects and figures into the toy house; hence, the verb was likely to be *擺 baai2* [put]. In response to the therapist's question about what to do, a typically developing child would use the verb *擺 baai2* [put] before the preposition *喺 hai2* [at] to make it clear where to put the television set. Without the verb, CY's sentence in [20] only states that the unspecified object is on the TV set. While there is no problem with grammar, the sentence does not communicate what was called for in the context.

[20]* *我知，喺哩X電視機度嘅。*
ngo5 zi1, hai2 le1 X din6si6gei1 dou6 ge3
I know, at INT X TV PRT SFP
(I know, (it's) placed on the TV set.)

[21] and [22] illustrate a Topic Comment structure in which the verb *擺 baai2* [put] after the Modal Auxiliary *可以 ho2ji5* [can] was omitted. Such an absence is syntactically acceptable in some discourse contexts – say, in response to questions for which the verb has been given. In the absence of such a context in which the two sentences were produced, the omission makes the meaning of the sentences vague and incomplete.

[21]* *另外一邊呢可以㗎。*
ling6ngoi6 jat1 bin1 le1 ho2ji5 gaa3
the-other one side PRT can SFP
((We) can put (it) on the other side.)

[22]* *上層呢唔可以㗎。*
soeng6 cang4 le1 m4 ho2ji5 gaa3
up deck PRT not can SFP
((We) cannot put (it) on the upper deck.)

b. Errors in incontiguous Serial Verb Constructions

As mentioned earlier, CY correctly produced four Serial Verb Constructions. They are of two semantic types: instrumental and purpose. Three of these four Serial Verb Constructions were of the contiguous type in which the verbs were chained together without an object noun between them. These contiguous Serial Verb Constructions develop earlier than the non-contiguous ones (Fung, 2011). CY was able to produce one non-contiguous Serial Verb Construction that was interrupted by an Interjection between the two verb phrases. CY made mistakes in two other attempts to produce a non-contiguous Serial Verb Construction.

[23] reveals both an argument omission and a word order error. While the patient (i.e., *面 min6* [face]) of the action *抹maat3* [wipe] could be dropped in a pragmatically appropriate context, its omission in this discourse context is inappropriate. In addition, placement of the verb *抹 maat3* [wipe] before the instrument object *毛巾 mo4gan1* [towel] required for the action is a syntactic violation. A typically developing child would produce a non-contiguous instrumental Serial Verb Construction like [24].

[23]* *跟住我要刷牙啦，*
gan1zyu6 ngo5 jiu3 caat3 ngaa4 laa1,
and-then I need-to brush teeth SFP,
跟住哩，我呢，抹哩毛巾啦。
gan1zyu6 le1, ngo5 le1, maat3 le1 mou4gan1 laa1
and-then INT, I PRT, wipe INT towel SFP
(Then I have to brush my teeth, and then I use a towel to wipe (my face).)

[24] *跟住我要刷牙啦，*
gan1zyu6 ngo5 jiu3 caat3 ngaa4 laa1,
and-then I need-to brush teeth SFP,
跟住我用毛巾抹面啦。
gan1zyu6 ngo5 jung6 mou4gan1 maat3 min6 laa1
and-then I use towel wipe face SFP
(Then I have to brush my teeth, and then I use a towel to wipe my face.)

[25] illustrates another instance of CY's problem with non-contiguous Serial Verb Constructions, this time of the purpose type. A typically developing child would use the verb *去 heoi3* [go] before *巴士站baa1si2zaam6* [bus stop] together with the other verb 玩waan2 [play] to make a grammatically appropriate and semantically complete Serial Verb Construction.

[25] INV: *去邊度玩呀?*
(Where do (we) go play?)
CHI: *我哋巴士站呀玩呀。*
ngo5dei2 baa1si6zaam6 aa1 waan2 aa3
we bus-stop INT play SFP
(We go to the bus stop to play.)

c. Errors in complex syntax

In addition to Serial Verb Constructions, CY also had difficulties indicating temporal relations in her sentences. CY's sentence in [4] does not include a Temporal Conjunction. [26] is grammatically inappropriate, with the absence of a temporal conjunction (e.g., *之後 zi1hau6* [after]) after the verb phrase 食完 *sik6 jyun4* [eat finish]. The temporal adverb *就 zau6* [then] before the verb *玩 waan2* [play] is also omitted in the sentence. A typically developing child would produce a sentence like [27].

[26]* *不如我哋食完呢我哋呢玩。*
bat1jyu4 ngo5dei2 sik6 jyun4 le1 ngo5dei2 le1 waan2
rather we eat finish PRT we PRT play
(Why don't we finish eating and then we play?)

[27] *不如我哋食完之後就玩囉。*
bat1jyu4 ngo5dei2 sik6 jyun4 zi1hau6 zau6 waan2 lo3
rather we eat finish after then play SFP
(Why don't we finish eating and then we play?)

[28] is an error sentence that involves both temporal and causal relations. While the causal relation could be left unmarked without the Conjunction *因爲 jan1wai6* [because], the temporal relation needs to be made explicit. A typically developing child would put the verb *食 sik6* [eat], together with the Verbal Particle *完 jyun4* [finish] and the Temporal Adverb *就 zau6* [then] before the Modal Auxiliary *可以 ho2ji5* [can] in the second clause as in [29].

[28]* *你要哩，快啲食哩，可以玩呀。*
nei5 jiu3 le1, faai3 di1 sik6 le1, ho2ji5 waan2 aa3
you need-to INT, quick a-bit eat INT, can play SFP
(You have to eat more quickly, so then (you) can play.)

[29] *你要快啲食，因爲食完就可以玩呀。*
nei5 jiu3 faai3 di1 sik6 jan1wai6 sik6 jyun4 zau6 ho2ji5 waan2 aa3
you need-to quick a-bit eat because eat finish then can play SFP
(You have to eat more quickly, because after (you) finish eating, (you) can play.)

CY's struggle with organizing her propositions into a meaningful and grammatically appropriate sentence or clause is made clear in [30]. The sentence is an attempt to answer the therapist's question on why we need to lock the door. The basic structure is a dependent clause that begins with the Causal Conjunction *因爲 jan1wai6* [because]. CY's adjective phrase *好快 hou2 faai3* [very quick] and the verb phrases *出現 ceot1jin6* [appear] and *行 haang1* [walk] are separated by an Interjection and are not connected in any way by other clausal elements or grammatical markers. With these phrases, the clause appears fragmented, and CY's intended propositions are made rather ambiguous. Another point to note is that CY uses the hand gesture of sneaking something from someone to complement her sentence. As an answer to the therapist's question, actually a simple clause expressing one proposition would suffice. A typically developing child would produce a clause like [31]. The clause includes a Pivotal Construction involving the verb *俾 bei2* [allow].

[30]* *因爲唔可以俾佢哩，人呢，好快哩，出現哩，*
jan1wai6 m4 ho2ji5 bei2 keoi5 le1, jan4 le1, hou2 faai3 le1, ceot1jin6 le1,
because not can allow him/her INT, person PRT, very quick INT, appear INT,
行哩XX係咁嘅偷嘢嘅。
hang4 le1 XX hai6 gam3 ge3 tau1 je5 ge3
walk INT XX be like-this SFP steal thing SFP
(Because (we) cannot allow him/her to appear quickly and steal from us like this.)

[31] *因爲唔可以俾佢偷嘢嘅。*
jan1wai6 m4 ho2ji5 bei2 keoi5 tau1 je5 ge3
because not can allow him/her steal thing SFP
(Because (we) cannot allow him/her to steal (from us).)

Despite these errors, as can be seen in Appendix B, CY was able to produce dependent clauses with the proper use of the Concession Conjunction *但係 daan6hai6* [but], the Temporal Conjunctions *跟住 gan1zyu6* [and then] and *然後 jin4hau6* [then] and the Causal Conjunction *因爲 jan1wai6* [because]. [32] shows the *然後 jin4hau6* [then], and [33] shows the *因爲 jan1wai6* [because] sentences. In both sentences, there were two Interjections.

[32] 然後哩，我要哩，洗手呀。
jin4hau6 le1 ngo5 jiu3 le1 sai2 sau2 aa3
then INT I need-to INT wash hand(s) SFP
(And then, I need to wash my hands.)

[33] *因爲你呢，有哩，人呢，開唔到依個㗎。*
jan1wai6 nei5 le1, jau5 le1, jan4 le1, hoi1 m4 dou2 ji1 go3 gaa3
because you PRT, have INT, person PRT, open not PRT this CL SFP
(Because some people cannot open this.)

d. Mazes and Interjections

As is clear in the discussion so far, CY's used mazes and Interjections often, particularly in her longer sentences. In [33], CY corrected herself and decided that the sentence subject was people rather than the therapist. In the same sentence, she produced one Interjection. In [34], CY produces a topic marker and one Interjection in the grammatically correct contiguous Serial Verb Construction. Having said that, many of CY's mazes and Interjections appear in grammatically inappropriate sentences, suggesting problems in sentence formulation. A typical example is seen in [30].

[34] *媽咪我呢，好早哩，去參觀呀。*
maa1mi1 ngo5 le1, hou2 zou2 le1, heoi3 caam1gun1 aa3
mommy I PRT, very early INT, go visit SFP
(Mommy, I go early to visit (the park).)

Appendix B also shows that CY did not produce any Passive Structures, *將 zeong1* Constructions or sentences with the *俾 bei2* [for]/[to] Preposition Phrase or the *對 deoi3* [to]/[towards] Prepositional Phrase. Complex Sentences without Overt Conjunctions were also not observed.

As an interim summary, we can conclude that CY sometimes omitted the verb in her sentences. Her production of non-contiguous Serial Verb Constructions was characterized by the omission of one of the component verbs and word order problems. CY had trouble with the formulation of sentences with temporal relations, particularly in the use of Temporal Conjunctions and Temporal Adverbs. This observation is consistent with To et al.'s (2010) observation of the problems school-age children with DLD have with the use of Conjunctions in narratives. CY's complex sentences with multiple propositions were often incomplete and interrupted by mazes and frequent Interjections.

Questions

CY asked three different types of Questions, although *wh* questions were not included.

Sentence Adverbs

Recall that Conjunctions were discussed early with Sentence Structures, and Sentence Final Particles were discussed in relation to language use. In terms of Sentence Adverbs, CY used one Temporal Adverb and one Frequency Adverb in her sentences.

4.5.4 Breakdown in the integration of language form, content and use

In the previous sections, language use, content and form were discussed as if they were unrelated. In actual moments of communication, they need to be properly integrated. Many of CY's errors, especially those involving more complex syntax, including Serial Verb Constructions and clauses with Temporal and Causal Conjunctions, reveal a breakdown in this integration because of inadequate knowledge and/or mastery of language form. Having said that, in [35], CY shows successful integration of language form, content and use during a role play with the toy figures.

[35]

INV: *坐低啦。*
Sit down.

CHI: *未得呀，問吓媽咪得未先呀。*
mei6 dak1 aa3, man6 haa5 maa1mi1 dak1 mei6 sin1 aa1
not-yet can SFP, ask ASP mommy ready yet first SFP
(Can't sit down yet. Let's ask Mommy if (she) is ready.)

INV: *好呀，你去問啦家姐。*
Okay. You go ask older sister.

CHI: *媽咪，得未呀？煮完未呀？煮完啦，*
maa1mi1, dak1 mei6 aa3? zyu2 jyun4 mei6 aa3? zyu2 jyun4 laa1
mommy, ready yet SFP? cook finish yet SFP? cook finish SFP
可以食早餐喇。
ho2ji5 sik6 zou2caan1 laa3
can eat breakfast SFP
(Mommy, are (you) ready? Have (you) finished cooking yet? (You) have finished cooking. We can eat breakfast.)

INV: 好呀。
Good.
CHI: 好呀。
hou2 aa3
good SFP
(Good.)

4.5.5 Summary

CY was a 6;4-old child with DLD. CY's primary problem was language form, although problems with language content in terms of vocabulary and definition were also an issue. An analysis of CY's language using the GACS framework revealed that she used a fairly diverse set of forms to modify her verbs, despite the presence of omission errors and inaccurate use of some forms in isolation or in combination with one another in some contexts. CY used the basic Sentence Structures productively. In addition, she was able to produce simple contiguous Serial Verb Constructions, sentences with Clausal Complements and clauses involving the use of some Conjunctions. Despite the diversity of Sentence Structures, many of CY's sentences revealed argument omission or other grammatical errors like word order. Often her sentences were interrupted by mazes and frequent Interjections. CY was also observed to use gestures to complement her speech occasionally. Having said this, there were forms and structures in all sections of the GACS that were not observed in CY's conversational sample. Conclusions cannot be drawn on these items as their absence could be a result of either CY's lack of knowledge or lack of opportunities in that particularly conversational context.

To conclude, CY was an interactive child with lots to talk about. Her ability to communicate effectively could be constrained by a number of different factors, including incomplete or inaccurate grammatical knowledge or unstable knowledge that could not be activated in time during sentence formulation, resulting in grammatical errors, mazes or frequent Interjections.

4.6 Five- and six-year-old children with DLD

One may ask if errors observed in the 6;4-old CY could also be seen in other children with DLD. To answer this question, we refer to conversational samples of two children with DLD in the Wong et al. (2010) corpus whose GACS scores were reported in Chapter 3. These two children were the closest in age to CY. They were the 5;7-old 20DLD and the 6;7-old 01DLD.

According to Table 3.9, on the basis of the HKU-70X samples, we learn that for Noun Phrase Expansion, children show productive use of Classifiers around the age of 3. For Verb Phrase Expansion, children show productive use of Modal Auxiliaries and Resultative Particles around the age of 4 and Aspect Markers around 4;6. For Sentence Structures, children show productive use of Serial Verb Constructions around the age of 4;6. Lastly, children show productive use of Temporal

Adverbs around the age of 4. As reported in the last section, at 6;4, CY demonstrated errors in the use of individual forms and structures in these word classes and sentence types at least some of the time. So we focus our attention on these forms and structures in the two children with DLD.

4.6.1 Noun Phrase Expansion

01DLD used the generic Classifier *個 go3* instead of the more specific Classifier *隻 zek3* for the noun *眼 ngaan5* [eye]. No omission or substitution errors were observed in 20DLD. It is important to note that while CY omitted the specific Classifier *張 zoeng1*, it was not a consistent error. In the conversation sample, CY was able to use the specific Classifier *道dou6* for door and the generic classifier *個 go3* appropriately.

4.6.2 Verb Phrase Expansion

While CY omitted the Aspect Marker *緊 gan2* in [16], 20DLD also omitted the Aspect Marker *咗 zo2* on one occasion. Before he produced sentence [36], 20DLD made two comments about the toy people that came with the house: there were a lot of people, and there were too many people. Therefore, in this context, it would be more appropriate to include the Aspect Marker *咗 zo2* as in [37]. In addition, the Classifier for quantity *啲 di1* [some] instead of *個 go3* should be used.

[36]* 多個人
do1 go3 jan4
more CL person
(one more person)

[37] *多咗啲人*
do1 zo2 di1 jan4
more ASP some person
(some more people than before)

In [38], 20DLD also used the Aspect Marker *咗 zo2* inappropriately. Given the context set up by the conditional conjunction *如果 jyu4gwo2* [if], the Modal Auxiliary *會 wui5* [will/would] for possibility should be used instead of the Aspect Marker *咗 zo2*. A typically developing child would produce a sentence like [39]. In fact, CY made a similar error in [12] discussed earlier. Note that the Conjunction *如果 jyu4gwo2* [if] often appears paired with the Conjunction *就 zau6* [then] to indicate conditional relations.

[38]* *如果佢一齊去燒燶咗 . . .*
jyu4gwo2 keoi5 jat1cai4 heoi3 siu1 lung1 zo2 . . .
if s/he together go burn burned ASP . . .
(If s/he goes together to get burned . . .)

[39] *如果佢一齊去就會燒燶 . . .*
jyu4gwo2 keoi5 jat1cai4 heoi3 zau6 wui5 siu1 lung1 . . .
if s/he together go then will burn burned . . .
(If s/he goes together, then s/he will get burned . . .)

4.6.3 Sentence Structures

CY was able to produce three contiguous Serial Verb Constructions. She was successful in one non-contiguous Serial Verb Construction but demonstrated grammatical errors in two of them, suggesting incomplete or incorrect knowledge. No errors in Serial Verb Constructions were noted in the two children with DLD. In fact, 20DLD produced one non-contiguous Serial Verb Construction of the purpose type, and 01DLD produced three instrumental and one benefactive Serial Verb Constructions, all of the non-contiguous type.

CY was able to produce two sentences with the *喺 hai2* [at] Prepositional Phrase. It was, however, not observed in 01DLD. 20DLD used it inappropriately in two questions and a sentence. In [40], 20DLD did not put in the preposition *喺 hai2* [at] between the noun and the where-question word. In [41], 20DLD substituted the preposition *喺 hai2* [at] with the Verb *瞓 fan3* [sleep], which came before the noun phrase *嗰個地下 go2 go3 dei6haa2* [that floor].

[40]* *哩雲邊度㗎？*
le1 wan4 bin1dou6 gaa3
INT cloud where SFP
(Where is the cloud?)

[41]* *我瞓嗰個地下瞓啦。*
ngo5 fan3 go2 go3 dei6haa2 fan3 aa3
I sleep that CL floor sleep SFP
(I sleep on the floor.)

4.6.4 Sentence Adverbs

As seen in Appendix B, CY used the Temporal Adverb *就 zau6* [then] correctly in one instance. But she also omitted it in [26] and [28] discussed earlier. In fact, CY demonstrated other problems with the proper expression of temporal relations in her sentences. 01DLD omitted the temporal adverb *就 zau6* [then] in [42] before the verb *做 zou6* [do]. The use of the Resultative Particle *完 jyun4* [finish], followed by the Temporal Adverb *就 zau6* [then] would make the temporal sequence of getting off school and doing homework more explicit.

[42]* *我放完學做㗎喇。*
ngo5 fong3-jyun4-hok6 zou6 gaa3 laa3
I release-school+finish do SFP SFP
(I do (it) after school is dismissed.)

4.6.5 Mazes and Interjections

Recall that CY produced mazes and Interjections often, making her sentences sound fragmented. The use of mazes was observed in [43], which was produced by 01DLD, and Interjection was observed in [44], which was produced by 20DLD. Neither of these children, however, produced mazes and Interjections to the extent that CY did.

[43] *<我今日個> [//]，我今日仲未擦嘅*
<ngo5 gam1jat6 go3> [//], ngo5 gam1jat6 zung6 mei6 caat3 ge2
< I today CL> [//], I today still not-yet brush SFP
(I have not yet brushed (it) today.)

[44] *因爲哩係俾細個啲人瞓，*
jan1wai6 le1 hai6 bei2 sai3go2 di1 jan4 fan3,
because INT be for small CL person sleep,
或者小朋友瞓㗎囉。
waak6ze2 siu2pang4jau5 fan3 gaa3 lo1
or little-kids sleep SFP SFP
(Because (this) is for those people who are young or little kids to sleep on.)

4.6.6 Summary

In this section, we examined the conversational samples from two children with DLD in the Wong et al. (2010) corpus who were the closest in age with CY. The goal was to see if some common grammatical features could be identified in five- to six-year-old Cantonese-speaking children with DLD. Not one grammatical form or structure was found to be problematic for these two children with DLD and CY. There were, however, forms and structures that were used inappropriately in one or two of these three children with DLD. Those observed in two children with DLD included Classifiers, for which one child produced a substitution and the other an omission error. The omission of Aspect Markers, the substitution of a Modal Auxiliary with an Aspect Marker and difficulties with markings of temporal relations such as Temporal Adverbs were observed in two children with DLD. Errors observed in one of the three children with DLD included non-contiguous Serial Verb Constructions and Sentences with the *喺 hai2* [at] Prepositional Phrase. Recall that at the beginning of Section 4.6, it was pointed out that all these forms and structures were reported to be used productively in the sample of 70 typically developing children before the age of 4;6 in the HKU-70X corpus.

Given a sample of only three children with DLD, we could not draw conclusions that the forms and structures reported in this chapter are potential clinical markers for DLD in Cantonese. Future research can examine these forms and structures using valid experimental tasks from a larger sample of children. Careful examination of children's errors in these tasks will also provide much needed insight into the nature of the difficulties Cantonese-speaking children with DLD have in language learning and use.

The report on the linguistic profile of CY in Section 4.5 and the report on the errors observed in two other five- to six-year-old children with DLD in Section 4.6 contributed to the existing literature on DLD, and DLD in Cantonese in particular. Like their English-speaking peers, Cantonese-speaking children with DLD also demonstrated problems in Verb Phrase Expansion, albeit of a difficult nature given that morphemes for modifying verbs in Cantonese are not inflectional. There are four plausible explanations for problems observed in Cantonese-speaking children with DLD's use of morphemes for Verb Phrase Expansion. First, these morphemes, including Modal Auxiliaries, Aspect Markers and Verbal Particles, are grammatically optional. Second, there are several different types and a substantial number of Verbal Particles in Cantonese. Third, many Verbal Particles and Aspect Markers have subtle distinctions in meaning, and they can appear together to modify verbs. Fourth, Modal Auxiliaries, Verbal Particles and Aspect Markers can be combined, and yet their combinations are determined on the basis of semantic compatibility rather than a paradigmatic structure.

The two reports also drew our attention to problems that Cantonese-speaking children with DLD have with grammatical constructions, including Serial Verb Constructions, Sentences with the 喺 *hai2* [at] Prepositional Phrase and complex sentences involving temporal relations.

4.7 Intervention goals for the 6;4 child with DLD using results from language sample analysis

In the long run, it will be helpful to identify all the language forms and structures that will successfully differentiate Cantonese-speaking children with DLD from their typically developing age peers at different stages of development. Once identified, these forms and structures can be used as clinical markers for the identification of DLD and considered high-priority intervention targets for children affected by it.

Before that day, how can we make decisions on intervention targets for individual children with DLD? In one of the first conceptual papers on language intervention, Johnston (1985) proposed three general principles: Fit, Focus and Functionality. While Focus is more relevant for the choice of intervention procedures, Functionality is related to activities. Fit is directly related to goal selection. A goal fits when it expresses the child's meanings and desired purposes. A goal fits when the child can understand it using his/her language knowledge and knowledge of the world.

For CY, ideally, it would be good to decide on intervention goals after considering the results of the grammatical analysis of her narrative sample and perhaps analysis of another sample collected during conversation on different topics. For the purpose of this exercise, we will only make use of information obtained from her conversational sample. CY had problems with vocabulary breadth and depth, as revealed in her word definitions. Vocabulary would be one of her goals. In this section, we will focus on her other goal: grammar.

One could first consider forms and structures that were not observed in her language samples. The challenge, however, is that while absence could be a result of lack of knowledge, it could also be due to the lack of opportunity. One could certainly identify forms and structures that were expected for her age and test her on them in criterion-referenced probes to confirm whether she actually did not have knowledge and hence required intervention. As mentioned in Chapter 2, current evidence on age of productive use of different grammatical forms and structures came only from the HKU-70X corpus, a relatively small cross-sectional sample of 70 Cantonese-speaking children between 2;5 and 5;8.

A more useful alternative is to examine CY's errors. Error patterns can reveal what language forms and structures she had difficulties with when talking about what she was interested in. Learning the forms or structures to meet her communication needs would fulfill the principle of Fit and would be highly motivating for her.

CY had problems in forms involving Verb Phrase Expansion and in Sentence Structures. Both would be a good fit for her. But which one should be on a higher priority? Generally speaking, we would choose Sentence Structures before Verb Phrase Expansion. This is because many forms for Verb Phrase Expansion are grammatically optional; hence, their omission might escape the notice of laypersons and would not draw much negative attention. The downside to this is that CY would not be able to express the nuanced meanings these forms provide in the verbs. On the other hand, the errors CY showed in Sentence Structures, like wrong word order, omission of essential clausal elements and frequent Interjections called much negative attention to her. Also, CY had a lot of ideas she wanted to share with others. Learning to use sentences properly would improve her communication competence in terms of both efficiency and effectiveness.

If Sentence Structures was the area to be considered for the grammar goal, which structure would CY be most ready to learn? Serial Verb Constructions would be a good choice. First of all, CY was already using the basic Sentence Structures, which provided the foundation for learning the more complex ones, including Serial Verb Constructions. Second, CY was also using the early-developing contiguous Serial Verb Constructions. Having said that, she produced these constructions with frequent Interjections. Therefore, initially, setting contiguous Serial Verb Constructions as a goal to help her develop automaticity in their production would be appropriate. Once this level was reached, CY would be ready to learn the non-contiguous Serial Verb Constructions of the instrumental or the purpose type as she made mistakes in one attempt at each of these types in the conversation. The choice would be confirmed after a few criterion-referenced baseline probes to see which one CY was more ready to learn given intervention. Given her obvious problem with sentence formulation, we should ascertain that CY reached a level of automatic production of the target non-contiguous Serial

Verb Construction in a variety of linguistic contexts and tasks before proceeding to the next goal.

Intervention goals could be determined on the basis of the results of a language sample analysis (Owens et al., 2018). In this section, we illustrated how we could do this using the GACS framework with a Cantonese-speaking child with DLD. While we paid attention to CY errors in the decision-making process, we also took note of what language forms and structures she already knew. Her existing knowledge would lay the foundation for subsequent learning of forms and structures that were more challenging to her.

4.8 Summary

This chapter reported on grammatical problems observed in Cantonese-speaking children with DLD through conversational analyses using the GACS framework. However, the use of the framework should not be restricted to children with DLD. It can be used to analyze conversational samples from children with language disorders in general, including those with language disorders associated with a biomedical condition, like intellectual disability or autism spectrum disorder. This chapter ended with an illustration of goal selection for a child with DLD on the basis of a grammatical analysis of her conversation sample. Again, the principle of Fit for goal selection should not be restricted to children with DLD. It can be applied to children with language disorders in general.

Notes

1 In the excerpts included in this chapter, for the sake of brevity, only the English translation is provided for the adult utterances in most circumstances. For child utterances, the English translation gives the child's meaning that is inferred from the context, whether or not the sentence is grammatically correct or semantically complete. INV stands for investigator. CHI stands for child.

2 * indicates unacceptable sentences with reference to the adult standard of use.

REFERENCES

Ambridge, B., & Lieven, E. V. M. (2011). *Child language acquisition: Contrasting theoretical approaches*. Cambridge University Press.

Bates, E., Dale, P. S., & Thal, D. (1995). Individual differences and their implications for theories of language development. In P. Fletcher & B. MacWhinney (Eds.), *The handbook of child language* (pp. 96–151). Blackwell Publishers.

Bates, E., & MacWhinney, B. (1982). Functionalist approaches to grammar. In E. Wanner & L. Gleitman (Eds.), *Language acquisition: The state of the art* (pp. 173–218). Cambridge University Press.

Bates, E., Thal, D., & MacWhinney, B. (1991). The functionalist approach to language and its implications for assessment and intervention. In T. M. Gallagher & C. A. Prutting (Eds.), *Pragmatics of language: Clinical practice issues* (pp. 133–161). Springer Publishing Group.

Berman, R. A., & Slobin, D. I. (1994). *Relating events in narrative: A crosslinguistic developmental study*. Lawrence Erlbaum Associates.

Bishop, D. V. M. (2014). Ten questions about terminology for children with unexplained language problems. *International Journal of Language and Communication Disorders, 49*(4), 381–415. https://doi.org/10.1111/1460-6984.12101

Bishop, D. V. M., Snowling, M. J., Thompson, P. A., & Greenhalgh, T. (2017). Phase 2 of CATALISE: A multinational and multidisciplinary Delphi consensus study of problems with language development: Terminology. *Journal of Child Psychology and Psychiatry, 58*(10), 1068–1080. https://doi.org/10.1111/jcpp.12721

Blake, J., Quartaro, G., & Onorati, S. (1993). Evaluating quantitative measures of grammatical complexity in spontaneous speech samples. *Journal of Child Language, 20*(1), 139–152. https://doi.org/10.1017/S0305000900009168

Bloom, L., & Lahey, M. (1978). *Language development and language disorders*. Wiley.

Brown, R. (1973). *A first language: The early stages*. Harvard University Press.

Census and Statistics Department, Hong Kong SAR Government (2007). *Population by*. www.censtatd.gov.hk/en/scode440.html

Census and Statistics Department, Hong Kong SAR Government (2017). *Population by census*. www.censtatd.gov.hk/en/scode459.html

Census and Statistics Department, Hong Kong SAR Government (2021). *Thematic household survey report No. 72*. www.censtatd.gov.hk/en/data/stat_report/product/C0000079/att/B11302722021XXXXB0100.pdf

Chan, A. W.-S. (2003). *The development of bei2 dative constructions in early child Cantonese*. Unpublished Master's Thesis. The Chinese University of Hong Kong.

Cheung, A. S.-Y. (1996). Acquisition of wh-words by Cantonese-speaking children. In T. H.-T. Lee, C.-H. Wong, S. Leung, P. Man, A. Cheung, K. Szeto, & C. S.-P. Wong (Eds.), *The development of grammatical competence in Cantonese-speaking children* (pp. 125–154). Report of a project funded by Hong Kong Research Grant Committee CUHK 2/91.

Cheung, C. C.-H., & Li, H. (2012). Outer and inner modifiers: The non-uniformity of *de* and *ge* in Mandarin and Cantonese. *Paper presented at the International Conference on Bilingualism and Comparative Linguistics*. The Chinese University of Hong Kong, May.

Cheung, P., Ng, A., & To, C. K.-S. (2006). *Hong Kong Cantonese articulation test*. City University of Hong Kong.

Cheung, S. H.-N. (2007). *A grammar of Cantonese as spoken in Hong Kong* (Rev. ed.) (in Chinese). The Chinese University of Hong Kong.

Child Assessment Service (2019). *Test of preschool oral language (Cantonese)*. Department of Health, Hong Kong SAR Government.

Clark, E. V. (2003). *First language acquisition*. Cambridge University Press.

Education Bureau (2008). *Pre-primary children development and behavior management: Teacher resource kit*. Hong Kong SAR Government. www.edb.gov.hk/en/edu-system/preprimary-kindergarten/comprehensive-child-development-service/index.html

Encyclopedia Britannica (n.d.). *Cantonese language*. www.britannica.com/topic/Cantonese-language

Ethnologue (2022). *What are the top 200 most spoken languages?* SIL International. www.ethnologue.com/guides/ethnologue200

Fletcher, P. (1985). *A child's learning of English*. Basil Blackwell.

Fletcher, P., Leonard, L. B., Stokes, S. F., & Wong, A. M.-Y. (2005). The expression of aspect in Cantonese-speaking children with specific language impairment. *Journal of Speech, Language, and Hearing Research*, *48*(3), 621–634. https://doi.org/10.1044/10924388(2005/043)

Fletcher, P., Leung, S. C.-S., Stokes, S. F., & Weizman, Z. (2000). *Cantonese pre-school language development: A guide*. Hong Kong Standing Committee on Language Education and Research.

Fletcher, P., & O'Toole, C. (2016). *Language development and language impairment: A problem-based introduction*. Wiley Blackwell.

Frank, M. C., Braginsky, M., Yurovsky, D., & Marchman, V. A. (2017). Wordbank: An open repository for developmental vocabulary data. *Journal of Child Language*, *44*(3), 677–694. https://doi.org/10.1017/S0305000916000209

Fung, R. S.-Y. (2000). *Final particles in standard Cantonese: Semantic extension and pragmatic inference*. Unpublished Doctoral Dissertation. Ohio State University.

Fung, R. S.-Y. (2009). Characteristics of Chinese in relation to language disorders. In S. P. Law, B. S. Weekes, & A. M.-Y. Wong (Eds.), *Language disorders in speakers of Chinese* (pp. 1–18). Multilingual Matters.

Fung, S. S.-H. (2011). *The emergence of serial verb constructions in child Cantonese*. Unpublished Master's Thesis. The University of Hong Kong.

Heep Hong Society (1995). *Child development guide* (in Chinese). Heep Hong Society.

Hong Kong SAR Government (2021). *Hong Kong the facts: Education*. www.gov.hk/en/about/abouthk/factsheets/docs/education.pdf

Goldberg, A. E. (2006). *Constructions at work: The nature of generalization in language*. Oxford University Press.

Johnston, J. R. (1985). Fit, focus and functionality: An essay on early language intervention. *Child Language Teaching and Therapy*, *1*(2), 125–134.

Johnston, J. R. (2001). An alternate MLU calculation: Magnitude and variability effects. *Journal of Speech, Language, and Hearing Research*, *44*(1), 156–164. https://doi.org/10.1044/1092-4388(2001/014)

Kidd, E., & Garcia, R. (2022). How diverse is child language acquisition research. *First Language*. Advance Online Publication https://doi.org/10.1177/01427237211066405

Klee, T., Schaffer, M., May, S., Membrino, I., & Mougey, K. (1989). A comparison of the age-MLU relation in normal and specifically language-impaired preschool children. *Journal of Speech and Hearing Disorders*, *54*(2), 226–233. https://doi.org/10.1044/jshd.5402.226

Klee, T., Stokes, S. F., Wong, A. M.-Y., Fletcher, P., & Gavin, W. (2004). Utterance length and lexical diversity in Cantonese-speaking children with and without specific language impairment. *Journal of Speech, Language, and Hearing Research*, *47*(6), 1396–1410. https://doi.org/10.1044/1092-4388(2004/104)

Kwok, H. (1984). *Sentence particles in Cantonese*. Centre of Asian Studies, University of Hong Kong.

Language Explorer (2021). *Language analysis for healthcare and research*. www.languageexplorer.app/

Law, A. (2001). A-not-A questions in Cantonese. In C. Iten & A. Neeleman (Eds.), *UCL working papers in linguistics 13* (pp. 295–318). University College London.

Law, S.-P. (1990). *The syntax and phonology of Cantonese sentence-final particles*. Unpublished Doctoral Dissertation. Boston University.

Lee. T. H.-T. (1994). A Cantonese child language corpus. *The Chinese University of Hong Kong, Faculty of Arts, Humanities Bulletin*, *3*, 62–68.

Lee, T. H.-T. (1996). Focus adverbs in child Cantonese. In T. H.-T. Lee, C.-H. Wong, S. Leung, P. Man, A. Cheung, K. Szeto, & C. S.-P. Wong (Eds.), *The development of grammatical competence in Cantonese-speaking children* (pp. 84–106). Report of a project funded by Hong Kong Research Grant Committee CUHK 2/91.

Lee, T. H.-T., Wong, C.-H., Leung, S., Man, P., Cheung, A., Szeto, K., & Wong, C. S.-P. (Eds.) (1996). *The development of grammatical competence in Cantonese-speaking children*. Report of a project funded by Hong Kong Research Grant Committee CUHK 2/91.

Lee, T. H.-T., Wong, C. H., & Wong, C. S. P. (1996). Functional categories in child Cantonese. In T. H.-T. Lee, C.-H. Wong, S. Leung, P. Man, A. Cheung, K. Szeto, & C. S.-P. Wong (Eds.), *The development of grammatical competence in Cantonese-speaking children* (pp. 155–173). Report of a project funded by Hong Kong Research Grant Committee CUHK 2/91.

Leonard, L. B. (2014). *Children with specific language impairment* (2nd ed.). MIT Press.

Leonard, L. B., Deevy, P., Miller, C., Rauf, L., Charest, M., & Kurtz, R. (2003). The use of grammatical morphemes reflecting aspect and modality by children with specific language impairment. *Journal of Child Language*, *30*(4), 769–795. https://doi.org/10.1017/s0305000903005816

Leonard, L. B., Deevy, P., Wong, A. M.-Y., Stokes, S. F., & Fletcher, P. (2007). Modal verbs with and without tense: A study of English- and Cantonese-speaking children with specific language impairment. *International Journal of Language and Communication Disorders*, *42*(2), 209–228. https://doi.org/10.1080/13682820600624240

Leonard, L. B., Wong, A. M.-Y., Deevy, P., Stokes, S. F., & Fletcher, P. (2006). The production of passives by children with specific language impairment acquiring English or Cantonese. *Applied Psycholinguistics, 27*(2), 267–299. https://doi.org/10.1017/S0142716406060280

Leung, C. S. (1995). *The development of aspect markers in a Cantonese-speaking child between the ages of 21 and 45 months*. Unpublished Doctoral Dissertation. University of Hawaii.

Leung, M.-T., & Li, H.-L. (2016). Cantonese LARSP: A procedure for assessment and remediation for Cantonese-speaking children. In P. Fletcher, M. J. Ball, & D. Crystal (Eds.), *Profiling grammar: More languages of LARSP* (pp. 172–197). Multilingual Matters.

Li, D. C. S. (2006). Chinese as a lingua Franca in greater China. *Annual Review of Applied Linguistics, 26*, 149–176. https://doi.org/10.1017/S0267190506000080

Li, H., Tse, S.-K., Wong, J. M.-S., Wong, E. C.-M., & Leung, S. O. (2013). The development of interrogative forms and functions in early childhood Cantonese. *First Language, 33*(2), 168–181. https://doi.org/10.1177/0142723713479422

Linguistic Society of Hong Kong (1997). *The Cantonese romanization scheme* (in Chinese). Linguistic Society of Hong Kong.

Luke, K.-K. (1990). *Utterance particles in Cantonese conversation*. John Benjamins.

Luke, K.-K., & Bodomo, A. (2001). A comparative study of the semantics of serial verb constructions in Dagaare and Cantonese. *Language in Contrast, 3*(2), 165–180.

MacWhinney, B. (2000). *The CHILDES project: Tools for analyzing talk* (3rd ed.). Lawrence Erlbaum Associates.

Man, P. (1996). The realization and omission of subject and object in early Cantonese. In T. H.-T. Lee, Wong, C.-H., Leung, S., Man, P., Cheung, A., Szeto, K., and Wong, C. S.-P. (Eds.), *The development of grammatical competence in Cantonese-speaking children* (pp. 107–124): Report of a project funded by Hong Kong Research Grant Committee CUHK 2/91.

Matthews, S. (2006). On serial verbs in Cantonese. In Y. Alexandra Aikhenvald & R. M. W. Dixon (Eds.), *Serial verb constructions: A cross-linguistic typology* (pp. 69–87). Oxford University Press.

Matthews, S., & Yip, V. (1994). *Cantonese: A comprehensive grammar*. Routledge.

Matthews, S., & Yip, V. (2011). *Cantonese: A comprehensive grammar* (2nd ed.). Routledge.

Matthews, S., & Yip, V. (2017). Noun-modifying clauses in Cantonese. In Y. Matsumoto, B. Comrie, & P. Sells (Eds.), *Noun-modifying clause constructions in languages of Eurasia: Rethinking theoretical and geographical boundaries* (pp. 105–120). John Benjamins.

Miller, J. F. (1981). *Assessing language production in children: Experimental procedures*. University Park Press.

Miller, J. F., & Chapman, R. S. (1981). The relation between age and mean length of utterance in morphemes. *Journal of Speech and Hearing Research, 24*(2), 154–161. doi: 10.1044/jshr.2402.154

Nippold, M. A. (2021). *Language sampling with children and adolescents: Implications for intervention*. Plural Publishing.

Norbury, C. F., Gooch, D., Wray, C., Baird, G., Charman, T., Simonoff, E. . . . Pickles, A. (2016). The impact of nonverbal ability on prevalence and clinical presentation of language disorder: Evidence from a population study. *Journal of Child Psychology and Psychiatry, 57*(11), 1247–1257. https://doi.org/10.1111/jcpp.12573

Opper, S. (1996). *Hong Kong's young children: Their early development and learning*. The Hong Kong National Report, Part 2, of the first phase of the Pre-primary Project of the International Association for the Evaluation of Educational Achievement (IEA). The University of Hong Kong.

Owens, R. E., Pavelko, S. L., & Bambinelli, D. (2018). Moving beyond mean length of utterance: Analyzing language samples to identify intervention targets. *Perspectives of the ASHA Special Interest Groups, 3*(1), 5–22. https://doi.org/10.1044/persp3.SIG1.5

Packard, J. L. (2000). *The morphology of Chinese: A linguistic and cognitive approach*. Cambridge University Press.

Plante, E., Swisher, L., Kiernan, B., & Restrepo, M. A. (1993). Language matches: Illuminating or confounding? *Journal of Speech, Language, and Hearing Research, 36*(4), 772–776. https://doi.org/10.1044/jshr.3604.772

Reynell, J., & Huntley, M. (1987). *Reynell developmental language scales: Cantonese version*. NFER-Nelson.

Rice, M. L., Smolik, F., Perpich, D., Thompson, T., Rytting, N., & Blossom, M. (2010). Mean length of utterance levels in 6-month intervals for children 3 to 9 years with and without language impairments. *Journal of Speech, Language and Hearing Research, 53*(2), 333–349. https://doi.org/10.1044/1092-4388(2009/08-0183)

Rice, M. L., Wexler, K., & Hershberger, S. (1999). Tense over time: The longitudinal course of tense acquisition in children with specific language impairment. *Journal of Speech, Language, and Hearing Research, 41*(6), 1412–1431. https://doi.org/10.1044/jslhr.4106.1412

Salt Software LLC (2021). *Systematic analysis of language transcripts (SALT)*. www.saltsoftware.com/

Scarborough, H. S. (1990). Index of productive syntax. *Applied Psycholinguistics, 11*(1), 1–22. https://doi.org/10.1017/S0142716400008262

Scarborough, H. S., Rescorla, L., Tager-Flusberg, H., Fowler, A. E., & Sudhalter, V. (1991). The relation of utterance length to grammatical complexity in normal and language-disordered groups. *Applied Psycholinguistics, 12*(1), 23–45. https://doi.org/10.1017/S014271640000936X

Shi, D., & Huang, C.-R. (2016). Syntactic overview. In C.-R. Huang & D. Shi (Eds.), *A reference grammar of Chinese* (pp. 14–66). Cambridge University Press.

Simons, G. (2022). *Welcome to the 25th edition of Ethnologue*. www.ethnologue.com/ethnoblog/gary-simons/welcome-25th-edition

Sio, J. U.-S. (2006). *Modification and reference in the Chinese nominal*. Unpublished Doctoral Dissertation. Universiteit Leiden.

Stokes, S. F., & Fletcher, P. (2000). Lexical diversity and productivity in Cantonese-speaking children with specific language impairment. *International Journal of Language & Communication Disorders, 35*(4), 527–541. https://doi.org/10.1080/136828200750001278

Stokes, S. F., & Fletcher, P. (2003). Aspectual forms in Cantonese children with specific language impairment. *Linguistics, 41*(2), 381–405. https://doi.org/10.1515/ling.2003.013

Stokes, S. F., & So, L. K. H. (1997). Classifier use of language disordered and age-matched Cantonese speaking children. *Asia Pacific Journal of Speech, Language and Hearing, 2*, 83–101.

Szeto, K. (1996). Classifiers in Cantonese-speaking children from 1 year 5 months to 3 years 8 months. In T. H.-T. Lee, C.-H. Wong, S. Leung, P. Man, A. Cheung, K. Szeto, & C. S.-P. Wong (Eds.), *The development of grammatical competence in Cantonese-speaking children* (pp. 1–25). Report of a project funded by Hong Kong Research Grant Committee CUHK 2/91.

Tam, C. W. Y., & Stokes, S. F. (2001). Form and function of negation in early developmental Cantonese. *Journal of Child Language, 28*(2), 373–391. https://doi.org/10.1017/S0305000901004688

Tang, S.-W. (2015). *Lectures on Cantonese grammar* (in Chinese). Hong Kong Commercial Press.

Tardif, T., Fletcher, P., Zhang, Z.-X., & Liang, W.-L. (2008). *User's guide and manual for the Chinese communicative development inventories*. Peking University Medical Press.

To, C. K.-S. (2006). *Use of reference in Cantonese narratives: A developmental study*. Unpublished Doctoral Dissertation. University of Hong Kong.

To, C. K.-S., Stokes, S. F., Cheung, H.-T., & T'sou, B. (2010). Narrative assessment for Cantonese-speaking children. *Journal of Speech, Language and Hearing Research, 53*(3), 648–669. https://doi.org/10.1044/1092-4388(2009/08-0039)

To, C. K.-S., Stokes, S. F., Man, Y., & T'sou, B. (2013). An analysis of noun definition in Cantonese. *Language and Speech, 56*(Prt 1), 105–124. https://doi.org/10.1177/0023830912440794

Tomasello, M. (2003). *Constructing a language: A usage-based theory of language acquisition*. Cambridge University Press.

Tomblin, J. B., Records, N. L., Buckwalter, P., Zhang, X., Smith, E., & Obrien, M. (1997). Prevalence of specific language disorders in kindergarten children. *Journal of Speech, Language, and Hearing Research, 40*(6), 1245–1260. https://doi.org/10.1044/jslhr.4006.1245

Tse, S.-K. (Ed.). (2006). *Oral language development for preschool children in Hong Kong* (in Chinese). Hong Kong University Press.

Tse, S.-K., Chan, C., Kwong, S.-M., & Li, H. (2002). Sex differences in syntactic development: Evidence from Cantonese-speaking pre-schoolers in Hong Kong. *International Journal of Behavioral Development, 26*(6), 509–517. https://doi.org/10.1080/01650250143000463

Tse, S. K., & Li, H. (Eds.). (2011). *Early child Cantonese: Facts and implications*. De Gruyter Mouton.

Tse, S.-K., Li, H., & Leung, S.-O. (2007). The acquisition of Cantonese classifiers by preschool children in Hong Kong. *Journal of Child Language, 34*(3), 495–517. https://doi.org/10.1017/S0305000906007975

T'sou, B., Lee, T. H.-T., Tung, P., Man, Y., Chan, A., To, C. K. S., . . . Chan, B. B.-W. (2006). *Hong Kong Cantonese oral language assessment scale*. City University of Hong Kong.

van der Lely, H., & Battell, J. (2003). Wh-movement in children with grammatical SLI: A test of the RDDR hypothesis. *Language, 79*(1), 153–181. https://doi.org/10.1353/lan.2003.0089

Voniati, L., Armositis, S., & Tafiadis, D. (2021). Language sampling practices: A review for clinicians. *Evidence-Based Communication Assessment and Intervention, 15*(1), 24–45, https://doi.org/10.1080/17489539.2021.1920118

Wells, G. (1985). *Language development in the preschool years*. Cambridge University Press.

Wells, G. (1986). *The meaning makers: Children learning language and using language to learn*. Heinemann Educational Books.

Wong, A. M.-Y. (2022). *A narrative sample and a completed analysis using the GACN framework*. Unpublished Manuscript. the University of Hong Kong. www.dldchinese.com

Wong, A. M.-Y., Au, C. W.-S., & Stokes, S. (2004). Three measures of language production for Cantonese-speaking school-age children in a story-retelling task. *Journal of Speech, Language, and Hearing Research, 47*(5), 1164–1178. https://doi.org/10.1044/10924388(2004/086)

Wong, A. M.-Y., Cheung, C. C.-H., Lo, J. M.-W., & Wan, E. K.-H. (2021a). *A summary score sheet template for the Grammatical Analysis of Cantonese Samples* (GACS). Unpublished Manuscript. Faculty of Education, The University of Hong Kong. www.dldchinese.com

Wong, A. M.-Y., Cheung, C. C.-H., Lo, J. M.-W., & Wan, E. K.-H. (2021b). *A framework for the Grammatical Analysis of Cantonese Samples* (GACS). Unpublished Manuscript. Faculty of Education, The University of Hong Kong.

Wong, A. M.-Y., Cheung, C. C.-H., Lo, J. M.-W., & Wan, E. K.-H. (2022). *A framework for the Grammatical Analysis of Narrative Samples (GANS) and a summary score sheet template*. Unpublished Manuscript. Faculty of Education, The University of Hong Kong. www.dldchinese.com

Wong, A. M.-Y., Chow, D. C.-C., McBride-Cheng, C., & Stokes, S. F. (2010). Optional elements and variant structures in the productions of *bei2* "to give" dative constructions in Cantonese-speaking adults and three-year-old children. *Journal of Child Language, 37*(1), 175–196. https://doi.org/10.1017/S0305000909009416

Wong, A. M-Y., & Johnston, J. R. (2004). The development of discourse referencing in Cantonese-speaking children. *Journal of Child Language, 31*(3), 633–660. https://doi.org/10.1017/S030500090400604X

Wong, A. M.-Y., Klee, T., Stokes, S. F., Fletcher, P., & Leonard, L. B. (2010). Differentiating Cantonese-speaking pre-school children with and without SLI using MLU and lexical diversity (D). *Journal of Speech: Language and Hearing Research, 53*(3), 794–799. https://doi.org/10.1044/1092-4388(2009/08-0195)

Wong, A. M.-Y., Leonard, L. B., Fletcher, P., & Stokes, S. F. (2004). Questions without movement: A study of Cantonese-speaking children with and without specific language impairment. *Journal of Speech, Language, and Hearing Research, 47*(6), 1440–1453. https://doi.org/10.1044/1092-4388(2004/107)

Wong, A. M.-Y., Ng, A. K.-H., Cheung, J. S.-C., & Lam, J. P.-Y. (2021). *Diagnostic terminology for child language disorders in Chinese*. Unpublished Manuscript. Hong Kong Association of Speech Therapists.

Wong, C. (1998). First auxiliaries and modality in child Cantonese. In S. Matthews (Ed.), *Studies in Cantonese linguistics*. Linguistic Society of Hong Kong.

Wong, C.-H. (1996). The acquisition of *bei2* as verb and preposition in a Cantonese-speaking child. In T. H.-T. Lee, C.-H. Wong, S. Leung, P. Man, A. Cheung, K. Szeto, & C. S.-P. Wong (Eds.), *The development of grammatical competence in Cantonese-speaking children* (pp. 65–83). Report of a project funded by Hong Kong Research Grant Committee CUHK 2/91.

Wong, C. S.-P. (1996). The development of noun phrase structure in Cantonese-speaking children around two. In T. H.-T. Lee, C.-H. Wong, S. Leung, P. Man, A. Cheung, K. Szeto, & C. S.-P. Wong (Eds.), *The development of grammatical competence in Cantonese-speaking children* (pp. 26–64). Report of a project funded by Hong Kong Research Grant Committee CUHK 2/91.

Wong, L.-Y. (2002). *The morphology, syntax, and semantics of adverbs in Cantonese*. Unpublished Master's Thesis. The University of Hong Kong.

Wong, R. K.-S. (2004). The acquisition of polysemous forms: The case of *bei2* ("give") in Cantonese. In O. Fischer, M. Norde, & H. Perridon (Eds.), *Up and down the cline: The nature of grammaticalization* (pp. 325–343). John Benjamins.

Wong, W., & Ingram, D. (2003). Question acquisition by Cantonese-speaking children. *Journal of Multilingual Communication Disorders, 1*, 148–157.

Yip, V., & Matthews, S. (2006). Assessing language dominance in bilingual acquisition: A case for mean length utterance differentials. *Language Assessment Quarterly, 3*(2), 97–116. https://doi.org/10.1207/s15434311laq0302_2

Yip, V., & Matthews, S. (2007). *The bilingual child: Early development and language contact*. Cambridge University Press.

Zhan, W., & Bai, X. (2016). Sentence types. In C.-R. Huang & D. Shi (Eds.), *A reference grammar of Chinese* (pp. 401–450). Cambridge University Press.

ABBREVIATIONS

ADV	adverbial marker
ASP	aspect marker
CL	noun classifier
CONJ	conjunction
DEG	degree expression
INT	interjection
NEG	negation marker
ONO	onomatopoeic sound
POSS	possessive marker
PREP	preposition
PRT	particle
SFP	sentence final particle

APPENDIX A

@Begin
@Languages: cantonese
@Participants: INV Investigator, CHI Target_Child
@ID: cantonese|change_corpus_later|INV||female|||Investigator|||
@ID: cantonese|change_corpus_later|CHI||female|||Target_Child|||
@Group of CHI: DLD
@Coder: YY
@Birth of CHI:
@Date: 25–8–2017
@Location: KTC 3/F
@Time duration: 00:00–19:03
@Comment: child is 6;4 years of age
@Situation: CHI and INV were playing with the doll house.

⋆INV: 嘩!我今日呢度呢, 有間 + . . .
⋆CHI: 屋.
⋆INV: 係呀! 有間屋喎.
⋆INV: 咁而家呢,我呢, 想請你同我一齊呢, 擺啲傢私入去先.
⋆INV: 睇吓. 間屋裡面呢有張 + . . .
⋆CHI: 床.
⋆INV: 係呀. 床要嚟做咩㗎?
⋆CHI: 擺喺度.
⋆INV: 好呀. 咁要嚟做咩㗎, 張床?
⋆CHI: 我哋呢, 夜晚呢, 係呢, 瞓教嘅.
⋆INV: 係呀.好呀. 咁夜晚瞓教. 唔, 好呀.
⋆INV: 擺上面呢度夠晒安靜呀.
⋆INV: 瞓教嘅時候呢, 就瞓得好舒服啦.
⋆CHI: XX 喺度呀.

*INV: 不過我哋擺好晒啲嘢先請佢出嚟啦. 咦! 依個係 + . . .
*INV: [pointing to the sofa]
*CHI: 彈嘅.
*INV: 哦. 我知啦. 你梗係平時喺度咁樣彈嘅. [=laughter]
*CHI: 坐低嘅.
*INV: 坐低嘅. 咁呢個係 + . . .
*CHI: 挨住嘅.
*INV: 係呀. 挨住嘅.
*CHI: 呢個x挨住.
*INV: 呢個係梳化.
*CHI: 梳化.
*INV: 有大. 又有 + . . .
*CHI: 細.
*INV: 咁一人擺一張啦. 你擺邊張呀?
*CHI: [=pointing to the larger sofa]
*INV: 你擺大梳化. 我擺細梳化.
*INV: 擺邊度好呢?
*CHI: 呢度.
*INV: 好呀. 擺下層.
*INV: 好喎. 我個細梳化擺你側邊啦.
*CHI: 但係有人喺度㗎喎.
*INV: 係喎. 有人喺度喎.
*INV: 咁呀. 我擺另一邊啦.
*CHI: 但係依度門呢, 撞咗人呀.
*INV: 係喎. 咁點算呀?
*CHI: 我知. 喺呢x電視機度嘅.
*CHI: 係喺呢度.
*INV: 哦. 擺上層.
*CHI: 係.
*INV: 好啦.
*CHI: 望吓呢出邊嘅.
*INV: 又可以望到出面睇風景.
*INV: 幾好喎你個設計.
*INV: 好啦. 仲有呢, 攞依個 . . .
*INV: 哈哈 . . . 唔, 餐臺同埋凳.
*INV: 餐臺同凳攞嚟做咩呀?
*CHI: 攞嚟呢食嘢嘅.
*INV: 唔, 食嘢. 睇緊啲廚房先.
*CHI: 喺呢度.
*INV: 下面. 好呀. 擺下邊.
*INV: 你又幫我擺呀!
*CHI: 但係 . . . XX 門呢 XX 㗎喎.
*INV: 咁呀. 咁點算呀?
*CHI: 有火中間嗰個囉XX. 喺衣度先呢得嘅.
*INV: 呢度呢喺個火爐旁邊. 啱啱好呀.

*INV: 好嘢. 一張凳夠唔夠呀?
*CHI: 唔夠.
*INV: 咁 . . . 要多幾多張呀?
*INV: 要多幾多張呀?
*CHI: 三.
*INV: 要三張呀.
*INV: 搵吓先. 一. 二. 三.
*CHI: [=shook her head]
*INV: 三張呀唔啱咩?
*CHI: 唔啱.依個好大凳嘅. 塞唔到落去呀.
*INV: 係喎. 咁我再搵.
*INV: 咁你要 . . . 你攞住嗰兩張先啦!
*INV: 我再搵.
*INV: 呀. 好嘢. 我搵到啦.
*CHI: 係呀.
*INV: 啱晒啦依三張. 啱啱好呀.
*INV: 屋企仲有啲嘢好緊要㗎.
*CHI: 廁所.
*INV: 你屋企有冇呀?
*CHI: 有.
*INV: 點解咁緊要呀? 因爲 . . .
*INV: 我哋呢平時呢要去廁所啦. 要去洗手啦. 所以呢. 屋企呢一定要依樣嘢㗎.
*INV: 咁而家我就攞喺 . . . 上層.
*CHI: 上層呢唔可以㗎.
*INV: 點解呀?
*CHI: 因爲你呢, 有呢, 人呢開唔到依個㗎.
*INV: 哦. 哦. 因爲攞呢度會阻住開唔到個櫃.
*INV: 咁攞呢邊啦. 呢邊?
*CHI: 唔好呀. xx人行, 有人行呢跌咗落去㗎.
*INV: 咁下邊啦. 下邊啦. 下邊. 好唔好啲呀?
*CHI: 好啲. 但係呢有道門呢撞咗呢呢個人呢.
*INV: 咁另外一邊啦.
*CHI: 另外一邊呢可以㗎.
*INV: 好啦. 咁就呢邊啦.
*INV: 加多一樣嘢先.
*INV: 你睇吓. 我有+ . . .
*INV: 哎呀跌咗. 哎呀又再跌咗.
*INV: 咩嚟㗎?
*CHI: 燈.
*INV: 係呀. 有燈呀.
*CHI: 喺呢呢度嘅燈.
*INV: 好呀. 攞喺睡房度.
*INV: 要嚟做咩嘢呀?

*CHI: 我哋呢要呢瞓教呢要熄燈嘅.
*INV: 哦. 瞓教要熄燈.
*INV: 咁平時要嚟做咩㗎?
*CHI: 要嚟呢. 係開燈呢抹眼鏡.
*INV: 係呀. 幾時要開燈呀?
*INV: 幾時開呀?
*CHI: 係六點鐘.
*INV: 係喎. 朝頭早六點定夜晚六點鐘呀?
*CHI: 八點鐘.
*INV: 哦. 八點鐘.
*INV: 黑 mang1 mang1 夜晚黑定係朝頭早呀?
*CHI: 朝頭早.
*INV: 朝頭早呀?
*INV: 好似而家咁樣呀?
*INV: 有啲地方呢, 朝頭早都開燈嘅.
*INV: 不過通常屋企呢夜晚黑呀夜晚先開燈.
*INV: 臨瞓前好似你咁講啱啦. 就熄咗盞燈.
*INV: 好啦. 差唔多啦.
*INV: 我差啲唔記得咗呀. 依張床俾BB 架.
*CHI: BB 嚟嘅.
*INV: 係呀俾BB 瞓㗎.
*CHI: 呢喺呢度瞓㗎.
*INV: 係呀. 係咪好似妹妹咁呀?
*CHI: 係.
*INV: 咁妹妹瞓喺邊度呀?
*CHI: 瞓喺床度嘅.
*INV: 係囉. 你幫我帶佢返屋企呀.
*INV: 妹妹張床擺喺 . . . 廁所度.
*CHI: 唔好.
*INV: 擺喺 . . . 廚房度.
*CHI: 唔好. 就擺喺度先.
*INV: 擺喺睡房度.
*CHI: 係.
*INV: 好啦. 我哋擺咗啲傢私啦.
*INV: 我哋而家呢, 準備帶佢玩啦喎.
*INV: 你睇吓. 屋度有 + . . .
*CHI: 爸爸. 媽咪.
*INV: 係呀. 有爸爸啦. 有媽咪啦. 仲有 + . . .
*CHI: 細佬.
*INV: 仲有 + . . .
*CHI: 姐姐. 細佬. BB.
*INV: 呀係呀. 佢哋一家人呢喺屋企好開心呀.
*INV: 等我睇吓先.
*INV: 睇吓媽咪做咩先.

*INV: 媽咪呢. 媽咪呢朝頭早呢, 起身啦喎, 就去廚房度整早餐.
*INV: 跟著呢攞喺臺面到先.
*INV: 然後呢, 哎呢度. 然後呢. 媽咪去嗌BB起身啦.
*INV: BB, 起身啦. 哥哥, 起身啦. 然後呢, 媽咪呢, 就 . . .
*CHI: 掉轉咗呀你.
*INV: 係咩. 哦. 咁樣啦. 然後呢媽咪就抱BB喎. 帶BB去廁所.
*INV: 跟著呢再帶BB 呢坐低. 然後一齊食早餐.
*CHI: 佢自己㗎喎.
*INV: 哎呀. 跌親添.
*CHI: 唔係呀. 自己㗎.
*INV: 要自己呀. 邊個要自己呀?
*CHI: 係XX 我哋呢自己學㗎.
*INV: 學自己食早餐.
*CHI: 係呀.
*INV: 好叻喎. 咁你睇吓.
*INV: 姐姐做咩呀?
*CHI: 起身.
*INV: 你帶佢呀.
*INV: 家姐做咩呀?
*INV: 家姐同媽咪. 好呀.
*CHI: 媽咪.
*INV: 咩事呀?
*CHI: 我要食早餐.
*INV: 好呀. 你想食咩嘢呀?
*CHI: 飯. 菜. 雞.
*INV: 咩話? 你再講多次.
*CHI: 飯. 雞. 菜.
*INV: 嘩! 咁多嘢呀.
*CHI: 係呀.
*INV: 你今日呢咁好胃口.
*INV: 好啦. 我去廚房度煮先.
*INV: 你自己玩吓先啦. 等一陣喎.
*CHI: 佢去廁所啦.
*INV: 好呀. 佢去廁所啦. 帶佢去呀.
*CHI: 好啦. xx準備去廁所啦.
*INV: 好喎.
*CHI: XX 好啦. 痾 wi1 wi1 啦.
*CHI: 我痾完啦.
*CH: 我沖廁所先.
*INV: 好呀. kam2 埋個廁所板.
*CHI: 跟住呢. 我沖咗.
*INV: 沖咗啦. 然後點呀?
*CHI: 然後呢我要呢洗手呀.
*INV: 係呀. 好叻呀. 又記得洗乾淨隻手喎.
*CHI: 跟著我要刷牙啦.

*CHI: 跟著呢, 我呢, 抹呢毛巾啦.
*INV: 抹乾淨隻手.
*CHI: 我得啦媽咪.
*INV: 哦. 我都差唔多整好啦.
*INV: 而家整緊雞呀. 蒸雞呀. 仲要呢炒菜.
*INV: 你玩一陣先啦.
*CHI: 好.
*INV: 好呀. 你去睇吓妹妹呀.
*CHI: 好. 妹妹你呢同我一齊玩啦.
*INV: 好呀. 姐姐. 姐姐我哋玩咩嘢呀?
*CHI: 哥哥呢瞓教呀. 我哋叫佢呢一齊玩呀.
*INV: 哦, 好呀. 我跟住你呀.
*CHI: 你拖住我啦.
*INV: 拖住. 都好乖喎. 我跟住你.
*INV: 拖住行. 上樓梯.
*CHI: 哥哥起身啦, 佢係融啦.
*INV: 咩事呀?
*CHI: 哎呀未呀. 咁樣起身.
*INV: 哦. 咩事?
*CHI: 我哋開始玩啦.
*CHI: 我哋好肚餓啦.
*INV: 去邊度玩呀?
*CHI: 我哋巴士站呀玩呀.
*INV: 跳 XX.
*INV: 去巴士站玩呀?
*INV: 但我聞到媽咪就嚟整好晚餐啦.
*INV: 我聞到啲晚餐香味喎.
*CHI: 不如我哋食完呢我哋呢玩囉.
*INV: 哦. 咁都好喎. 我哋落去食飯先.
*CHI: 好.
*INV: 家姐. 等埋我呀.
*CHI: 我等你.
*INV: 家姐等埋呀.
*CHI: 好啦. 我哋呢食嘢啦開始.
*CHI: 開凳先.
*INV: 坐低啦.
*CHI: 未得呀. 問吓媽咪得未先呀.
*INV: 好呀. 你去問啦家姐.
*CHI: 媽咪. 得未呀?
*CHI: 煮完未呀?
*CHI: 煮完啦. 可以食早餐啦.
*INV: 好呀.
*CHI: 好呀.
*INV: 我坐 . . . 我坐呢邊.
*CHI: 唔好呀. 呢個BB架跌咗架 (13:52).

*INV: 我坐 . . . 臺上面.
*CHI: 唔好呀. 會跌架.
*INV: 哎呀. 我跌到個頭好痛呀.
*CHI: 我呢要呢坐呢度㗎哥哥.
*INV: 哦. 知道. 好啦.
*CHI: BB 我抱你上去啦.
*INV: 好呀. 家姐抱. 家姐抱BB.
*CHI: 好呀. 呢度.
*INV: 小心呀.
*INV: 係喎. BB 你坐得好好喎.
*CHI: 哥哥.
*INV: 係.
*CHI: 坐低啦.
*INV: 係. 我嚟啦嚟啦. 嚟啦嚟啦.
*INV: 坐. 我坐BB 隔籬.
*CHI: 我坐呢. 媽咪隔籬.
*INV: 好喎. 媽咪整好飯啦.
*INV: 媽咪整好早餐.
*CHI: BB 跌咗呀.
*INV: 係呀. 媽咪攞早餐出嚟呀.
*INV: 你幫我帶媽咪呀.
*INV: 我攞早餐出嚟.
*CHI: 好呀. 我呢攞早餐.
*INV: 媽咪話. 你哋 + . . .
*CHI: 你哋呢. OK 呀.
*INV: 好呀. 你哋呢. 慢慢食.
*CHI: 我OK 呀.
*INV: 慢慢食.
*CHI: 慢慢食呀. 知唔知呀?
*CHI: 你要呢, 快啲食呢, 可以玩呀. 知唔知呀?
*INV: 哦.
*CHI: 知道呀媽咪.
*CHI: 媽咪呢好肚餓.
*INV: 媽咪都好肚餓.
*INV: 係呀. 媽咪話 . . . 媽咪呢 . . . 個個媽咪都係咁架. 成日提小朋友. 快啲食啦. 食完可以 玩啦.
*INV: 咁呢. 媽咪又坐好啦.
*CHI: 爹地呢?
*INV: 媽咪呢第一個食完啦.
*INV: 哦. 爹地出嚟啦. 爹地出嚟啦.
*CHI: 呢度呀呢度.
*CHI: 我入嚟啦.
*INV: 爹地早晨.
*CHI: 早晨哥哥.

*INV:	爹地早晨.
*CHI:	早晨姐姐.
*INV:	爹地早晨.
*CHI:	早晨BB.
*CHI:	喂. 媽咪我呢, 好早呢, 去呢參觀呀.
*CHI:	啊.
*CHI:	到我玩啦真係. XX 係呀. XX.
*INV:	係呀. 好呀. 咁我哋呢.
*CHI:	呢度呀.
*INV:	呢邊又參觀呀.
*INV:	好呀. 咁呢我哋帶埋小朋友一齊去啦.
*CHI:	我哋一齊去啦. 人呢要出去呢玩囉. 好喎.
*INV:	好呀. 哎呀. 家姐嚟啦. 爹地爹地. 哥哥嚟啦. 家姐. 爹地. 媽咪. 我嚟啦.
*CHI:	好呀.
*CHI:	你又會跌架BB.
*INV:	等埋我.
*CHI:	BB 嚟架, 唔得㗎BB.
*INV:	咁應該點呀?
*CHI:	爹地爹地! XX 我抱你啦. 好.
*INV:	好.
*CHI:	好呀.
*CHI:	XX 我哋行啦. 好喎.
*INV:	好喎. 我哋去參觀啦.
*CHI:	Yeah.
*INV:	喺邊到架?
*CHI:	喺屋企嘅 XX 囉. 櫃囉.
*INV:	哦. 好呀. 一齊行啦. 依邊. 係咪呀?
*CHI:	唔係呀. XXX
*INV:	哦. 好. 我行啦. 我出去禁lift 呀.
*INV:	快啲同我一齊. 禁lift. 禁lift.
*INV:	好. 閂門. 閂門. 叮. 閂 門. 鎖門.
*CHI:	鎖門.
*INV:	點解要鎖門呀?
*CHI:	因爲唔可以俾佢呢, 人呢, 好快呢, 出現呢, 行呢XX係咁嘅偷嘢嘅.
*INV:	哦.係呀,唔好俾人偷嘢呀.
*INV:	好. 鎖好門啦. 我哋行啦.
*CHI:	Yeah.
*INV:	Yeah.
*CHI:	係呢度啦.
*INV:	好啦. 我哋唔好嘈佢哋參觀啦.
*INV:	我哋收埋. 我哋就玩第二樣玩具啦.
*INV:	佢哋入去參觀啦. bye bye.
@End

APPENDIX B

Summary of analysis on CY using the GACS framework

A. Noun phrase expansion (NP)

		Exemplar 1	*Exemplar 2*	*Exemplar 3*	*Exemplar 4*
Cl	***1. Classifiers***	. . . 依<u>道</u>門 . . .	. . . 呢<u>個</u>人 . . .		
Poss	***2. Possessive constructions***	呢個<u>BB架</u> . . .			
Adj Mod	***3. Adjectival modifiers***	. . . 依個好<u>大</u>凳嘅			
Nom Mod	***4. Nominal modifiers***				
Loc Mod	***5. Locative modifiers***				
Prep Mod	***6. Prepositional modifiers***	<u>喺屋企嘅 XX</u> 囉, <u>櫃囉</u>	. . . <u>喺呢呢度嘅燈</u>		
RC	***7. Relative clauses***				

6/28

B. Verb phrase expansion (VP)

		Exemplar 1	*Exemplar 2*	*Exemplar 3*	*Exemplar 4*
Aux	***1. Auxiliaries***	. . . 要呢瞓教呢	可以食早餐啦	會跌架	
Mod Aux	1.1 Modal auxiliaries				
Oth Aux	1.2 Other auxiliaries				
V Adv	***2. Verbal adverbs***				
Man Adv	2.1 Manner Adverbs	妹妹你呢同我一齊玩啦	慢慢食呀	快啲食呢	好快呢, 出現呢
Neg Adv	2.2 Negation Adverbs	唔夠	未得呀		
Deg Adv	2.3 Degree Adverbs	我哋好肚餓啦			
Asp	***3. Aspect markers***	挨住嘅	掉轉咗呀您	問吓媽咪 . . .	
VPrt	***4. Verbal particles***				
Res Prt	4.1 Resultative particles	塞唔到落去呀	掉轉咗呀你	我痾完啦	
Dir Prt	4.2 Directional particles	BB 我抱你上去啦	我入嚟啦	塞唔到落去呀	坐低啦
Pot Prt	4.3 Potential particles	人呢開唔到依個架.			
Oth VPrt	4.4 Other verbal particles				
Comp	***5. Complements***				
Des Comp	5.1 Descriptive complements				
Ext Comp	5.2 Complements of extent				
Loc Comp	*5.3 Complements of location*				
Loc	5.3.1 Localizers	我坐呢媽咪隔離	我呢要呢坐呢度架哥哥	望吓呢出邊嘅	
PP	5.3.2 Prepositional phrases	擺喺度	瞓喺床度嘅		

C. Sentence structures (SS)

		Exemplar 1	*Exemplar 2*	*Exemplar 3*	*Exemplar 4*
VO	***1. Verb-object structure***	痾 wil wil	係六點鐘	鎖門	
SVO	***2. Subject-verb-object structure***	我要食早餐	佢去廁所啦	我沖廁所先	你拖住我啦
SV	***3. Subject-verb structure***	我知	我痾完啦	我得啦媽咪	我入嚟啦
SA	***4. Subject-adjective structure***	我哋好肚餓啦	我OK 呀	媽咪呢好肚餓	
SN	***5. Subject-noun structure***				
Top	***6. Topic structure***				
EC	***7. Existential constructions***	但係有人喺度架喎	xx 人行有人行呢	但係呢有道門呢撞咗呢呢個人呢	
Com C	***8. Comparative constructions***				
Com A	8.1 Comparison of adjectives	**好啲**			
Com Qua	8.2 Comparing quantities				
PC	***9. Pivotal constructions***	我哋叫佢呢一齊玩呀			
Pass	***10. Passive structure***				
ZC	***11. Zoeng1 construction***				

S PP	***12. Sentences with a prepositional phrase***				
	12.1 *bei2* construction				
	12.2 hai2 construction	呢**喺**呢度瞓架	**喺**依度先呢得嘅		
	12.3 *deoi3* construction				
	12.4 *tung4* construction	妹妹你呢**同**我一齊玩啦			
	12.5 *dou3* construction	**到**我玩啦			
CC	***13. Clausal complements***	問吓**媽咪得未先**呀	我地開始**玩**喇	XX 準備**去廁所**喇	
SVC	***14. Serial verb constructions***				
	14.1 Simple SVC-1	**攞**嚟呢**食**嘢嘅	. . . 人呢要**出**去呢**玩**囉	媽咪我呢，好早呢，**去參觀**呀	係**開**燈呢**抹**眼鏡
	14.2 Complex SVC-2				
CS-Conj	***15. Complex sentences without overt conjunctions***				

Section Score: 30/100

D. Questions (Q)

		Exemplar 1	*Exemplar 2*	*Exemplar 3*	*Exemplar 4*
YN	***1. Yes/No questions***				
Prt Q	1.1 Particle questions	爹地呢?			
A Q	1.2 A-not-A questions				
Cop Q	1.3 Copula questions				
Mei6 Q	1.4 Mei6 questions	得未呀?	煮完未呀?		
Exi Q	1.5 Existential questions				
Tag Q	1.6 Tag questions	慢慢食呀, 知唔知呀?			
Int Q	1.7 Intonation questions				
Ech Q	1.8 Echo questions				
WhQ	***2. Wh questions***				
					4/40

E. Sentence adverbs, conjunctions and sentence final particles

		Exemplar 1	*Exemplar 2*	*Exemplar 3*	*Exemplar 4*
S Adv	***1. Sentence adverbs***				
Sco Adv	1.1 Scope adverbs				
Tem Adv	1.2 Temporal adverbs	就擺喺度先			
Fre Adv	1.3 Adverbs of frequency	你又會跌架BB			
Mod Adv	1.4 Modal adverbs				
Conj	***2. Conjunctions***				
Coor Conj	2.1 Coordinating conjunctions				
Caus Conj	2.2 Cause conjunctions	因爲你呢, 有呢, 人呢開唔到依個架			
Conc Conj	2.3 Concession conjunctions	但係有人喺度架喎			
Cond Conj	2.4 Conditional conjunctions				
Temp Conj	2.5 Temporal conjunctions	跟著我要刷牙啦	然後呢我要呢洗手呀		
Purp Conj	2.6 Purpose conjunctions				
SFP	***3. Sentence final particles***	瞓教嘅 我哋一齊去啦人呢要出去呢玩囉	XX 喺度呀 好喎	但係有人喺度架喎 唔好. 就擺喺度先.	坐低啦 跟著呢

14/48

F. Errors

	Exemplar 1	*Exemplar 2*	*Exemplar 3*	*Exemplar 4*	*Exemplar 5*
1. Addition					
2. Omission	我知, (擺) 喺呢x電視機度嘅	哥哥呢馴(緊) 教呀	我哋(去) 巴士站呀玩呀	不如我哋食完 (之後) 呢, 我哋呢玩囉	你要呢, 快啲食呢, (食完就) 可以玩呀
	另外一邊呢可以(擺)㗎	佢(要)自己(食早餐)架喎	依個好大(張)凳嘅	上層呢唔可以(擺)㗎	有火(喺)中間嗰個囉
	(拉)開(張)凳先	我等(埋)你			
3. Wrong choice of words [4]	但係依道門呢, 撞咗(到)人呀	望吓(到)呢出邊嘅	呢個BB架(會)跌咗架	(會)撞咗(到)人呀	
4. Wrong order of words [3]	依個(凳)好大凳嘅	我呢, 抹呢毛巾啦			
5. Sentence formulation [3]	xx大行 有人行呢跌咗落去架	因爲你呢, 有呢, 大呢(會)開唔到依個架	因爲唔可以俾佢呢, 大呢, 好快呢, 出現呢, 行呢XX係咁嘅偷嘢嘅	我哋呢夜晚呢係呢馴教嘅	我哋一齊去啦大呢要出去呢玩囉
	我哋呢要呢馴教呢要熄燈嘅	媽咪我呢, 好早呢, 去呢參觀呀. 到我玩啦真係. XX 係呀. XX			
6. Others [4]	哥哥起身啦. 佢係融啦				

For Product Safety Concerns and Information please contact our EU representative GPSR@taylorandfrancis.com
Taylor & Francis Verlag GmbH, Kaufingerstraße 24, 80331 München, Germany

www.ingramcontent.com/pod-product-compliance
Ingram Content Group UK Ltd.
Pitfield, Milton Keynes, MK11 3LW, UK
UKHW022314250926
475702UK00046B/789
9780367424183